Intermittent Fasting for Women Over 50

© Copyright 2021 by EMMA VOGEL - All rights reserved.

This document is geared towards providing exact and reliable information regarding the topic and issue covered. The publication is sold with the idea that the publisher is not required to render accounting, officially permitted, or otherwise, qualified services. If advice is necessary, legal, or professional, a practiced individual in the profession should be ordered.

From a Declaration of Principles which was accepted and approved equally by a Committee of the American Bar Association and a Committee of Publishers and Associations.

In no way is it legal to reproduce, duplicate, or transmit any part of this document in either electronic means or printed format. Recording of this publication is strictly prohibited, and any storage of this document is not allowed unless with written permission from the publisher. All rights reserved.

The information provided herein is stated to be truthful and consistent. In terms of inattention or otherwise, any liability, by any usage or abuse of any policies, processes, or directions contained within is the solitary and utter responsibility of the recipient reader. Under no circumstances will any legal responsibility or blame be held against the publisher for reparation, damages, or monetary loss due to the information herein, either directly or indirectly.

Respective authors own all copyrights not held by the publisher.

The information herein is offered for informational purposes solely and is universal as such. The presentation of the information is without a contract or any type of guarantee assurance.

The trademarks used are without any consent, and the publication of the trademark is without permission or backing by the trademark owner.

All trademarks and brands within this book are for clarifying purposes only and are owned by the owners, not affiliated with this document.

Intermittent Fasting for Women Over 50

5 SCIENCE-PROVEN SOLUTIONS TO DELAY AGING BY LOSING WEIGHT AND INCREASING ENERGY WITHOUT GIVING UP YOUR LIFESTYLE EVEN IF YOU WORK A 9 TO 5 JOB.

Emma Vogel

TABLE OF CONTENT

INTRODUCTION — 1
History of Fasting — 5
Advantage of Intermittent Fasting — 6
Fasting for Diabetes — 7
Fasting for Heart Health — 8
Who Should Not Fast? — 9

PART 1: THE DIET

CHAPTER 1
WHAT IS INTERMITTENT FASTING — 10

Intermittent Fasting and Time Restricted Eating — 10
Intermittent Fasting Is Not a Diet. It's an Eating Pattern — 10
Misconceptions — 14
Is Intermittent Fasting Right for Me? — 14

CHAPTER 2
HOW INTERMITTENT FASTING WORKS — 16

How Intermittent Fasting Affects the Brain — 19
How Intermittent Fasting Affects the Mitochondria — 22
How Intermittent Fasting Affects the Immune System — 24

CHAPTER 3
HOW EFFECTIVE IS INTERMITTENT FASTING — 25

Intermittent Fasting for the Weight Loss Process — 27
Intermittent Fasting for Preventing Diseases — 28
Intermittent Fasting for the Anti-Aging Process — 29
Intermittent Fasting Practiced for Therapeutic Benefits — 30
Intermittent Fasting for Better Mental Performance — 32
Intermittent Fasting for an Improved Physical Fitness — 33
Intermittent Fasting for Bodybuilding — 34

CHAPTER 4
INTERMITTENT FASTING AND KETOSIS — 37
How to Apply Cyclic Ketosis and Fasting? — 38

CHAPTER 5
BENEFITS — 43
Improved Mental Concentration and Clarity — 43
Longevity — 43
Improvement in Hormone Profile — 44
Reduces Inflammation — 44
Polycystic Ovarian Syndrome and Intermittent Fasting — 45
Lower the Risk of Diabetes — 46
Improve Muscle Health — 46
Boosted Energy — 47
Lessen Oxidative Stress — 48
Improve Mental Well-Being — 49
Heart's Health — 50
Cellular Repair — 50
Boosts Your Immune System — 51
Improved Sex Drive — 51
Cellular Repair — 52

CHAPTER 6
SUCCESS STORIES — 53

CHAPTER 7
5 BEST METHODS OF INTERMITTENT FASTING FOR WOMEN OVER 50 — 62

Time-Restricted Eating (16:8 Method) — 63
The Twice-a-Week (5:2 method) — 65
Alternating Day Fasting — 66
Eat Stop Eat (24-Hour Fast) — 68
Spontaneous Meal Skipping — 69

PART 2: THE 14-DAY PROGRAM

CHAPTER 8
How to Start — 71
Get Clear on Your Goals — 71
Choose Your Method — 72
Identify Your Calorie Needs — 73
Conduct Meal Planning Without Overdoing It — 76
Begin Your IF Journey with the Pedal to the Metal — 78

CHAPTER 9
Mistakes to Avoid — 79
Making Lots of Changes within a Short Duration — 79
Not Monitoring Your Liquid Intake — 79
Not Drinking Adequate Water — 80
Feeding on Unhealthy Foods — 81
Overeating When You Break Your Fast — 81
Sticking with the Wrong Plan — 82

CHAPTER 10
Exercise to Do with Intermittent Fasting Diet — 83
Walking/Jogging — 85
Light Aerobics — 86
Stretching/Yoga — 86
Balance — 87

CHAPTER 11
Tips for Maintaining Intermittent Fasting — 88
Drinking Water and Organic Juices — 88

CHAPTER 12
What to Eat to Avoid Hungry Pains — 94
Water — 94
Fish — 95
Avocado — 95
Leafy Greens — 96

Potatoes	97
Probiotics	97
Assorted Berries	98
Eggs	98
Whole Grains	99
Legumes	99
Nuts	100

PART 3: MEAL PLAN

CHAPTER 13
THE 14-DAY GROCERY LIST — 101

Tips for Vegetable & Meat Selections	103
Example of How Meal Prep Works – The Shopping List	105
Method of Preparation	106

CHAPTER 14
THE 14-DAY RECIPES — 110

Breakfast		110
1	Smoked Salmon Omelet	110
2	Mushroom Scramble Egg	110
3	Matcha Green Tea Smoothie	111
4	Date and Walnut Porridge	112
Lunch		113
5	Asian Chicken Wings	113
6	Baked Garlic Ghee Chicken Breast	113
7	Lamb Curry	114
8	Healthy Baby Carrots	115
Dinner		116
9	Garlic Bread Stick	116
10	Steam Your Own Lobster	116
11	Garlic Ghee Pan-Fried Cod	117
Snacks		118
12	Orange and Apricot Bites	118
13	Zucchini Chips	118
14	Calamari Rings	119

CONCLUSION — 120

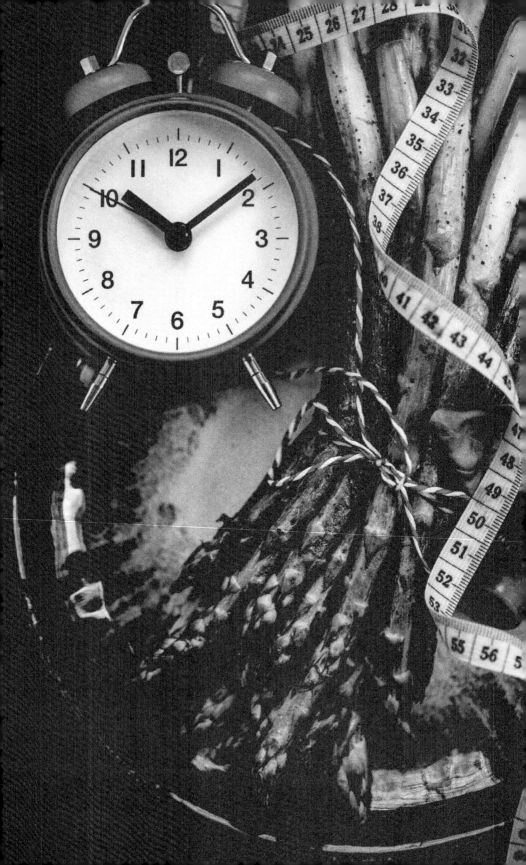

Emma Vogel

INTRODUCTION

Intermittent fasting (IF) is when you keep away any kind of foodstuff involving calories among ordinary nutritious ingredients. It is not starvation or a way for you to eat junk food with no consequences. There are various methods used to practice IF; they divide time into hours or divide time into days. Since the response to the regimen varies from person to person, no process can be called the best.

Intermittent fasting cannot make you lose those additional pounds instantaneously, but it can prevent unhealthy addictions. It's a nutritional practice that requires you to be determined to follow it and get the desired result. If you already have little time for eating due to your schedule, this regiment will suit you like a duck to water, but you will always need to be conscious of what you are eating. Choose the appropriate regiment after you take expert guidance. You should see it as a segment of your schedule to get healthy, but not the only component.

If you do it frequently, your body becomes used to it; thus, it automatically becomes a regular practice for you. Your body will alter your hunger patterns, as you'll feel famished when you're ready to eat rather than following false hunger signals. When intermittent fasting is done for more extended periods, it ends in quicker results, but long fasts are done less frequently. It is possible to switch plans, but don't do it because you find it hard initially, as all of them are quite similar.

Your eating patterns influence hormones that increase appetite and fat retention, like insulin. The quantity of food and the eating time affect your circadian rhythms. These circadian rhythms are predictable recurrent variations of hormone levels over a day—nearly all hormones, like those required for growth.

The circadian rhythms are affected by the season and time of the day. Food was most likely available during the day in the Paleolithic period, as they used the sunlight for hunting because they had no light source at night.

Other animals have inverted circadian rhythms because they hunt at night and sleep in the day. You may consume the same meals, but the timing can create a considerable variation in your body and general wellness. In the evening, the insulin levels are higher than in the morning, so eating large meals can cause more fat to be stored in your body. It helps connect the relationship between eating and obesity since it is more of a hormonal inequality than calorific inequality.

If you are in a heavily stressed environment, intermittent fasting can be challenging. It can do the opposite of what you want it to do as it can increase fat storage.

Believe it or not, a circadian rhythm was followed by hunger; otherwise, we would be hungry all the time. Need is lowest in the morning, and desire is at its highest at night. Hormones affect when you feel hungry, so the period you have stayed without eating doesn't matter. It takes time for hormones to adjust so that you may feel hungry during the first few days of fasting, but after that, you will not feel hungry during your time of fasting.

Many people say that breakfast is supposed to be the largest meal of the day, but in fact, you're the least hungry in the morning, as stated earlier. Eating a large breakfast is just forcing the body to eat food that it doesn't need; it hurts your weight loss goals. Your insulin concentrations are highest at night, leading to a lot of glucose converting into fat; thus, more fat is stored when you eat a large meal in the evening. Lunchtime is the optimum time to eat the largest meal of the day.

During a diet, burning up stored fats is the way the body gets energy. It will teach your body to use fats for strength and forfeit glucose, even when you're not fasting. In organs like the heart and lungs, your body utilizes stored fat for energy, but more is generated due to unnecessary eating. Also, organs using recycled fat do not have enough time to use that fat as glucose is carried continuously into the system, so the body first needs to get rid of it. If you eat a lot and do not exercise, your body cells cannot burn the stored fat.

By default, the cells of a healthy person are designed to burn fat for energy, so intermittent fasting is like adding gasoline to a fire. Encouraging your system to make fat—your only energy source—will help you lose more fat in the long run.

Exercise can help you with this process. Training allows your cells to consume fat and glucose when the body needs it, providing you energy rather than enhancing fat retention.

Emma Vogel

History of Fasting

According to the American Heart Association, intermittent fasting may be an effective way to lose weight, increase your metabolism, and increase longevity. This method involves periods of fasting that can range from 16 hours to 24 hours every day.

Although intermittent fasting is a new idea for most people, it certainly isn't a new concept. The most widely known version of it is called the "5:2 diet." In this diet, you eat 500 calories for some time, restricting your calorie intake to 500 calories for 2 days and then allowing yourself to eat up to 1,000 calories a day for the remaining 5 days.

Historically, humans have been doing intermittent fasting ever since they began eating food. There are many different kinds of fasting that have been practiced since ancient times. In some cases, minimal amounts of food or water were intermittently withheld from the body. For instance, when a person was in distress, fasting could provide spiritual and physical benefits. Many cultures still practice fasting worldwide today, such as in the Muslim world where laws require Muslims to fast at least once per year during Ramadan.

Advantage of Intermittent Fasting

There are a lot of advantages to intermittent fasting. First and foremost, it is a weight-loss method that allows you to eat whatever you want—within reason—while maintaining a healthy diet. You don't have to follow a strict exercise routine or count calories to lose weight. There are other benefits as well, such as increased energy, better mental clarity, and more! All you have to do is to learn how to do it properly.

It means that you don't have to skip meals to lose weight. You can eat all the food you want without any harm to your metabolism or health. Intermittent fasting is not difficult to learn if you follow the guide that we've provided.

But intermittent fasting isn't just about dropping pounds; it's also used to treat many other health conditions. Some examples include:

Insulin Resistance: One study found that fasting for people

who have insulin resistance can decrease insulin levels in the blood, improving their insulin sensitivity.

High Cholesterol: Intermittent fasting has been shown in studies to improve high cholesterol levels without any adverse effects on HDL (good cholesterol) levels. The study showed a decrease in total cholesterol and LDL (bad) cholesterol following an 8-week fast. Another study found four weeks of intermittent fasting increased HDL levels (good cholesterol) and decreased LDL levels.

Fasting for Diabetes

There are essential health benefits to intermittent fasting.

You may not be aware, but intermittent fasting has been used for centuries to reduce the risk of developing type II diabetes and other diseases.

You can do intermittent fasting by merely skipping meals. Studies have shown that this may play an essential role in reducing your heart disease risk, diabetes, cancer, and many other chronic diseases.

Some people like to fast by eating only from 9 a.m. and 3 p.m. Others prefer to fast for 16 hours, or from 6 p.m. until 11 p.m. The main thing is to try some different intermittent fasting schedules and see what works best for you.

Fasting for Heart Health

Fasting may be the only way to get all the ketogenic diet benefits without dietary restrictions. Intermittent fasting can help improve heart health, shed weight, and increase energy levels. Here's why: Intermittent fasting can help improve heart health because it increases your body's fat-burning potential by forcing the body to burn stored fat rather than glucose.

If your goal is to lose weight, intermittent fasting can lead to fewer calories consumed each day, potentially decreasing hunger and giving you more energy and focus throughout the day. It can also slash blood sugar levels, making it easier for you to maintain healthy blood sugar levels with less insulin resistance and a healthier metabolism.

Who Should Not Fast?

Some people should not fast. If you have a medical condition or are pregnant, please speak to a physician before starting a fast. Understand that fasting can cause more harm than good. Many people engage in intermittent fasting to control their weight, and so you could experience adverse side effects if you're not aware of them.

PART 1: THE DIET

CHAPTER 1
What Is Intermittent Fasting

Intermittent Fasting and Time Restricted Eating

Intermittent fasting is an eating pattern that will split your day into two periods: an eating period and a fasting period. This is why it is also called Intermittent Fasting and Time Restricted Eating.

Intermittent Fasting Is Not a Diet. It's an Eating Pattern

Intermittent Fasting was first introduced to the public in 2006 by Martin Berkhan, fitness veteran and author of the bestselling book The Leangains Method, but it started gaining incredible popularity only after celebrities like Hugh Jackman, Chris Hemsworth, Reese Witherspoon, Jennifer Aniston, and Kourtney Kardashian started talking about it. I am sure all of you may have seen the handsome Hugh Jackman talking about his rigid diet plan and the workout routine for the preparation of his movie Wolverine. In this interview, Hugh Jackman says that he could eat anything he wanted for 8 hours a day, and then he couldn't touch food for the following 16 hours.

Well... it was definitely worth it!

Intermittent fasting (IF) is an umbrella term for various eating schedule patterns with specific time intervals between consecutive meals.

I will show you the patterns in the next section, but for now we can say that there are two main ways to approach IF: strict and flexible. Strict IF involves fasting through the entire day, while flexible IF involves skipping meals or reducing calories on certain days of the week while keeping the overall calorie intake unchanged.

So, can you actually fast for so many hours a day?
How are you going to do it?
Aren't you going to feel hungry?
With food cravings?

Well, human fasting has actually been around for millennia.

Emma Vogel

Humans have been fasting since the beginning of the times. This is simply because in the old days, food was not always available, as it is today in our society. At least not for everyone!

Ancient Greeks, like Aristotle and Plato, supported fasting as a form of purification, and almost all religions include fasting as an element in their rituals. Therefore, we are perfectly capable of enduring fasting for a few hours. Don't worry, you will be fine.

In order to function through the day, your body needs glucose. Your body gets the glucose when you eat, in the carbohydrates that are broken down into glucose when you have a meal. This glucose is your main energy source. If you are on a high-carb or high-calorie diet, your body will store the extra energy as fat.

And this is not what we want.

So what happens with intermittent fasting?

The science behind intermittent fasting states that when you fast long enough your body will start accessing your fat reserves and you will start burning them. This allows your body to burn fat.

You can lower your fat and keep it off for good. You can lower your body fat and have a better figure. Improve your fitness and your health. Studies have shown that, while fat loss starts after 12 hours, it's after 16 hours that the benefit you're getting become exponential.

If you fast for less than 15 hours, it's going to give you benefits, but the difference that you can have between 17 and 15 is much bigger, thanks to the exponential effect.

Intermittent fasting may not be the right approach for everyone and as we will see through the book this is quite recent discovery. Nevertheless, study shows that intermittent fasting can lead to weight loss, fat burning, and a lot of other health benefits such as improving your brain's health and the lower your pressure and cholesterol.

Misconceptions

People always ask me: can I eat when fasting? Will I end up starving myself? Well, fasting is not a synonym for starving. I want you to understand that my goal is to help you find healthy and sustainable habits that will help you find joy and wellbeing. You will see how you will be able to enjoy food like never before and get the most benefits while doing it by modifying your eating patterns.

Intermittent fasting has the purpose of improving your life and your general health. I don't want you to start with preconceptions and think you won't be able to make it work, as I will do everything I can to show you how to introduce healthy habits in your life and get the results you deserve!

Is Intermittent Fasting Right for Me?

Intermittent fasting is not for everyone and I recommend you to consult your doctor or nutritionist if you want to start intermittent fasting.

Categories that should not fast are:

- Pregnant women
- Children or teens
- People that have eating disorders like for instance anorexia
- People with diabetes and other medical problems or people that are underweight.

CHAPTER 2
How Intermittent Fasting Works

Before we can fully grasp how intermittent fasting works, we must know that there are only two states in which the body can exist. Either the body is in the state of reserving food energy or utilizing or expending reserved energy. The primary goal of intermittent fasting is to ensure there is a balance in these two states.

Here is what happens during the fed state. When we consume food, the food goes through metabolism and then produces energy. Some of this energy is immediately spent, while some is reserved. The reservation of energy is a vital responsibility of a hormone called insulin. So, during the fed state (that is, the eating period), insulin increases to break down carbohydrates first into simple sugar units known as glucose. This glucose is what the body immediately converts into its fuel, which is known as adenosine triphosphate (ATP) — this process is known as catabolism.

Secondly, in order to store more energy, it then builds up glucose in glycogen, which is a more complex form of sugar. This process is known as anabolism. This built-up energy is stored in the liver, and sometimes muscles get broken down later into glucose (the form of energy the body can easily use). However, the body doesn't have an unlimited storage capacity to continue storing glycogen. So, what then happens when it hits its trench hold? The body initiates a process known as de-novo lipogenesis. This process is used to store more glucose by simply converting excess glucose into fat. In this form, the body has an unlimited storage capacity. Some of this newly converted fat could be stored in the liver, but a bulk of the fat is moved and stored all over the body. This is known as body fat, and it results in weight gain.

On the other hand, during the fasted state (that is, the period without eating), the body carries out the opposite process. The body reduces the production of insulin, which we know is responsible for the storage of energy. Once the insulin level drops, the body immediately knows its state has changed, and as such, its process must change.

Knowing full well there is no food coming in and hence no external source of energy, the body is forced to use its reserve. The body at this state begins to carry out catabolism. First, it starts breaking down glucose that was formerly stored in complex forms as glycogen.

The energy released in that process can sustain the body for up to 36 hours. If the body continues in this state, the body is further forced to start breaking down its fat reserve. This mode the body enters is called ketosis. It is the stage where the body switches from its usual and normal source of energy, which is glucose, to ketones and fat. With this, the body can have the energy to function for days depending on the amount of already accumulated fat. This process would result in weight loss naturally. When one intermittently fasts, they are only creating or maintaining the balance between the fed state and the fasted state. An imbalance may be in the side of always eating, which causes the body to have more calories than it really needs. Aside from that, it also continuously overworks the body as it continuously breaks down consumed food. This could result in several health issues. So, in order to remain healthy, one must, from time to time, frequently allow the body to use up its reserved energy. This is absolutely normal as all animals do it to maintain their health.

How Intermittent Fasting Affects the Brain

The brain is a vital organ responsible for controlling every other part of the body. And it will interest you to know that the human brain makes up less than 2% of the total body mass. It is the principal seat of intelligence and is responsible for our personal and societal developments. Among the numerous functions of the brain include; maintaining consciousness, memory recall, process data including languages, skill learning, and so on. So, the importance of ensuring that the necessary nutrients needed by the brain are provided cannot be overemphasized.

To keep the brain healthy and functioning at an optimal level, the brain uses up to about 20% of the calories generated each day. For such a small organ as the brain, one would think this amount of energy is too much. But the brain is always working, sending signals throughout the body. The signals sent by the brain either bring about voluntary actions or involuntary actions.

Even when we are asleep, the brain still works, although not as much as when we are wide awake.

If the brain needs this much energy to function, the next thing that might come to mind is that fasting would have a negative effect on it. But this is not true, as we will begin to examine how fasting works when it has to do with the brain. First of all, fasting plays a great role in the development of new brain cells.

When we intermittently fast, the brain-derived neurotrophic factor (BDNF) is triggered, facilitating the process of developing synapses and brain cells. Fasting also enhances serotonin, which is a chemical messenger in the brain. BDNF is commonly known to prevent stroke and depression. Fasting increases these functions and a lot more of BDNF up to about 55 to 350%.

Another way fasting affects the brain is it works to prevent neurodegeneration. We already know that fasting initiates autophagy, and during this process, beta-amyloid plaques are evacuated from the body, thus reducing oxidative stress, which might be on the neuronal tissue. Fasting has been reported to be one of the treatments for epileptic patients.

Intermittent fasting not only prevents degeneration but also enhances neuroregeneration and protection. This it does by boosting growth hormones, which act to prevent muscle depreciation. Lastly, fasting helps to facilitate mitochondrial biogenesis, which is known as the powerhouse of the cell.

The brain contains numerous cells and, as such, contains numerous mitochondria. A boost in mitochondria results in an increase of available energy in the brain. However, this will be discussed in detail below. Still, there is a wide range of beliefs that fasting causes starvation, leading to hypoglycemia.

This is the survival state of the body — instead of the body starting to convert saved glucose and subsequently stored fat in the body, the body continues to store up this energy and enters into a hibernation mode. At this stage, the blood sugar drops, and the body starts to shut down some of its functions.

The individual starts experiencing fatigue, shivers, low brain function in the form of forgetfulness, and lastly, fainting. While this might be true for extended unmonitored fasting, this is not the case for intermittent fasting. The reason is that one still eventually eats after avoiding food for some time. So, the body knows it has not gotten to starvation.

How Intermittent Fasting Affects the Mitochondria

Like we noted earlier, mitochondria are the powerhouse of the cells. Their health is very important to not only the cell but to the entire organism. To ensure the mitochondria (and the entire cell) remain in good health, dysfunctional cellular components eventually must be eliminated. Also, the cell needs to perpetually be in homeostasis, and free radicals, either chemicals or organelles, cannot be allowed to remain in the cell. All these processes can be triggered by time-controlled fasting.

Intermittent fasting can also engineer the development of new mitochondria through the process of mitochondria biogenesis. This process is a result of some metabolic regulators, which include AMPK and PGC-1. The regulators are responsible for not only building new mitochondria but also regulating mitophagy (the process where the mitochondria self-heals). They initiate the building of new mitochondria by sending signals to the body to increase the production of more energy in a stressful and energy-depleting environment (intermittent fasting). To follow this command, the cell then develops new mitochondria (power plants) to produce more energy. This process has the effect of keeping one always energized and youthful.

Intermittent fasting also boosts mitochondria density. This is the ability of the mitochondria to not just produce more energy while making use of fewer resources but to be very efficient in doing it. This development is a result of a boost in NAD+ levels, which is one function of intermittent fasting.

The NAD+ is an enzyme that plays a vital role for the mitochondria to be able to produce more energy. Its presence in the cell energizes the mitochondria in its early stages of life. It also restores and replenishes the mitochondria during old age. It does this by initiating mitophagy as well as DNA repair.

Another key function of the NAD+ is the activation of Sirtuins. Sirtuins are charged with the responsibility of protecting the cell from stress. Like we mentioned earlier, during intermittent fasting, the body begins to burn stored up body fat instead of its regular glucose. The breaking down of glucose leaves behind free radicals and produces higher oxidative stress when compared to breaking down fatty acids. So, we can say that intermittent fasting slows down mitochondria's aging process because it leads to the release of fewer free radicals and oxidative stress in the cell.

How Intermittent Fasting Affects the Immune System

The immune system is essential in the body as its health ensures the whole body's continued health. When fasting, stem cells are turned on.

These stem cells play vital roles in rejuvenating aging cells, which end up prolonging their youthfulness. An example of this stem cell is the Hematopoietic Stem Cell (HSC).

Fasting accomplishes this process by shutting down Cyclic Adenosine Monophosphate (cAMP) dependent Protein Kinase A (PKA). The cAMP is a molecule messenger, while PKA is a bunch of enzymes. Both are responsible for the regulation of fat, glycogen, and sugar metabolism.

Once PKA is shut down by turning on the cAMP signal, the body knows to start mobilizing its reserved energy. And the minute the body begins to burn body fat, stem cells are activated. But it takes time for this process to kickstart. This is because the body needs to finish burning all available glucose and all the glycogen it reserved before it can begin to burn body fat reserve. So, for this to happen, one has to engage in regular or long-term intermittent fasting. Also, fasting could act as stressors that could be harmful to the body. But if it is done correctly in time, it can become a handy tool. Gradually exposing the body to stressors through intermittent fasting helps the body get used to and develop resilience against them. So, the more one intermittently fasts, the more resilient to stressors one's immune system becomes.

CHAPTER 3
How Effective Is Intermittent Fasting

There are plenty of diets out there, all promising you the impossible. Incredible weight loss, with no mention of any side effects.

You are probably fed up with the "lose x pounds in 30 days, guaranteed" approach. Many of these diets are not backed up by science, or in other words, there is not any scientific research to prove these diets actually deliver what they promise. They focus only on the weight loss process, suggesting meal plans that are extremely radical in some cases. Diets mean nutrient deprivation in most cases, but they are plenty of cases when these diets have harmful effects on your health. Unlike other diets, focused on the weight loss process in an incredibly short amount of time, intermittent fasting is focusing more on your health, as nutritionists believe that health should be the most important factor, and only a healthy body can have a long and sustainable weight loss process. Unlike the other diets, which have a "hit and run" approach, IF is something for the long run and should be regarded as a way of life, not like a meal plan to be implemented for a few weeks. By checking out the benefits below, you can better understand why this process is so beneficial for your body.

The main benefits of intermittent fasting can be summarized in 8 points:

- Eliminates precancerous and cancerous cells
- Shifts easily into nutritional ketosis
- Reduces the fat tissue
- Enhances the gene expression for healthspan and longevity
- Induces autophagy and the apoptotic cellular repair or cleaning
- Improves your insulin sensitivity
- Reduces inflammation and oxidative stress
- Increases neuroprotection and cognitive effects

To expand on the benefits of this practice, intermittent fasting can have positive impacts on the fat loss process, disease prevention, anti-aging, therapeutic benefits (psychological, spiritual and physical), mental performance, physical fitness (improved metabolism, wind, and endurance, the great effect over bodybuilding).

Intermittent Fasting for the Weight Loss Process

As you restrain yourself from eating, the body will no longer have available glucose to use in order to produce energy.

Therefore, it will use ketones to break the fat tissue open and release the energy stored in there. This is how the body will burn your existing fat in order to generate energy. When it comes to diets, they are not designed for the long run, and as soon as you break the diet, you will start gaining weight again.

Intermittent fasting is something that you can try for a lifetime because it is easy to stick to it, and it doesn't involve any special meal plan. So, you can still eat your favorite foods, as long as you schedule your meals, allowing a smaller eating window and a longer fasting period.

IF induces ketosis and eventually autophagy, which will definitely mean reducing the fat reserves.

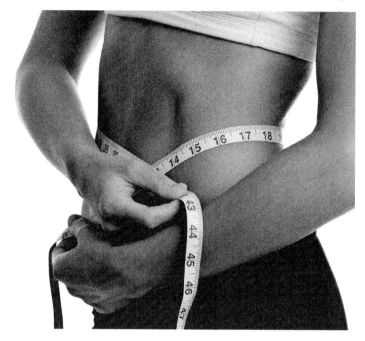

Intermittent Fasting for Preventing Diseases

What if you found out that intermittent fasting is, in fact, a cure for several different diseases and medical conditions? You would definitely become more interested in this process.

There are a few studies that show the beneficial effects IF has on your health. A study published in the World Journal of Diabetes has shown that patients with type 2 diabetes on short-term daily intermittent fasting experience a lower body weight, but also a better variability of post-meal glucose.

Other benefits this diet has are:

- Enhances the markers of stress resistance
- Reduces the blood pressure and inflammation
- Better lipid levels and glucose circulation, which may lead to a lower risk of cardiovascular disease, neurological diseases like Parkinson's and Alzheimer's, and also cancer

Intermittent Fasting for the Anti-Aging Process

The modern-day lifestyle includes too much stress and is too sedentary. Whether we like it or not, these factors have a great contribution to the aging process. You are probably wondering what intermittent fasting can do the slow down this process, as we all know that it can't be stopped. IF is not "the fountain of youth" and it will not grant you immortality, but it can still lower the blood pressure and reduce oxidative damage, enhance your insulin sensitivity and reduce your fat mass. Coincidence or not, all of these are factors are known to improve your health and longevity. Intermittent fasting is one of the triggering factors of autophagy, a process known for destroying and replacing old cell parts with new ones, at any level within your body. Such a

Emma Vogel

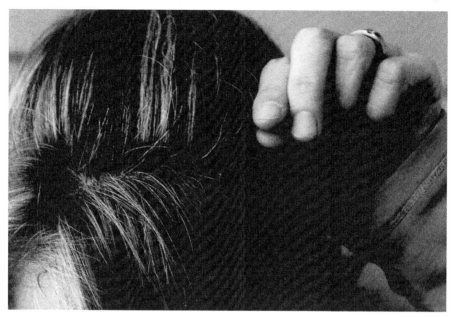

process can slow down the aging process.

Intermittent Fasting Practiced for Therapeutic Benefits

When it comes to therapeutic benefits, the most important ones are physical, spiritual and psychological.

In terms of physical benefits, intermittent fasting is a powerful cure for diabetes, but it can also prove to be very useful for reducing seizure-related brain damage and seizures themselves, but also for improving the symptoms of arthritis. This practice also has a spiritual value, as it's widely practiced for religious purposes across the globe. Although fasting is regarded as penance by some practitioners, it's also a practice for purifying your body and soul (according to the religious approach). Intermittent fasting is also about exercising control and will, over your body and your feelings. Achieving absolute control over your power and mind is a very powerful psychological benefit. You can ignore hunger, restrain yourself from eating for a certain period of time. In other words, IF is also associated with mind training and can also improve your self-esteem. A successful intermittent fasting regime can have very powerful effects from a psychological point of view. A study has shown that women practicing IF had amazing results in terms of senses of control, reward, pride, and achievement.

Intermittent Fasting for Better Mental Performance

IF also enhances the cognitive function and also is very useful when it comes to boosting your brainpower. There are several factors of intermittent fasting which can support this claim.

First of all, it boosts the level of brain-derived neurotrophic factor (also known as BDNF), which is a protein in your brain that can interact with the parts of your brain responsible for controlling cognitive and memory functions as well as learning. BDNF can even protect and stimulate the growth of new brain cells.

Through IF, you will enter the ketogenic state, during which your body turn fat into energy, by using ketones. Ketones can also feed your brain, and therefore improve your mental acuity, productivity, and energy.

Intermittent Fasting for an Improved Physical Fitness

This process influences not only your brain but also your digestive system. By setting a small feeding window and a larger fasting period, you will encourage the proper digestion of food. This leads to a proportional and healthy daily intake of food and calories. The more you get used to this process, the less you will experience hunger. If you are worried about slowing your metabolism, think again! IF enhances your metabolism, it makes metabolism more flexible, as the body has now the capability to run on glucose or fats for energy, in a very effective way. In other words, intermittent fasting leads to better metabolism.

Oxygen use during exercise is a crucial part of the success of your training. You simply can't have performance without adjusting your breathing habits during workouts. VO2 max represents the maximum amount of oxygen your body can use per minute or per kilogram of body weight. In popular terms, VO2 max is also referred to as "wind." The more oxygen you use, the better you will be able to perform.

Top athletes can have twice the VO2 level of those without any training. A study focused on the VO2 levels of a fasted group (they just skipped breakfast) and a non-fasted group (they had breakfast an hour before). For both groups, the VO2 level was at 3.5 L/min at the beginning, and after the study, the level showed a significant increase of "wind" for the fasting group (9.7%), compared to just 2.5% increase in the case of those with breakfast.

Intermittent Fasting for Bodybuilding

Having a narrow feeding window automatically mean fewer meals, so you can concentrate the daily calorie intake into just 1-2 consistent meals. Bodybuilders find this approach a lot more pleasing than having the same calorie consumption split into 5 or 6 different meals throughout the day. It's said that you need a specific amount of proteins just to maintain your muscle mass. However, muscle mass can be also maintained through intermittent fasting, a process which doesn't focus specifically on protein intake. Remember, the growth hormone reaches unbelievable levels after 48 hours of fasting, so you can easily maintain your muscles without eating many proteins, or having protein bars or shakes. As you already know, nothing is perfect and intermittent fasting is no exception. There are a few side effects that you need to worry about, like:

- Hunger is perhaps the most common side effect of this way of eating, but the more you get used to IF, the less hunger you will feel
- Beware of constipation, as when you eat less, you will not have to go to the toilet very often, so you can feel constipated at the beginning
- Headaches should be expected when fasting. Food deprivation is a direct cause of these headaches. However, controlling your hunger and getting used to fasting, will be

the best weapon to fight against these headaches

- During intermittent fasting, you might experience muscle cramps, heartburn, and dizziness
- In the case of athletic women, or those with very low body fat percentage, intermittent fasting may lead to a higher risk of irregular periods and lower chances of conception (so it reduces fertility for these women)

CHAPTER 4
Intermittent Fasting and Ketosis

The ketogenic diet offers many of the same benefits associated with intermittent fasting, and when done together, most people will experience significant health improvements, including not just weight loss. The ketogenic diet and intermittent fasting allow the body to move from a state where sugar is burned to a state where fat is burned (important flexibility, which in turn promotes optimal cell function and body systems). And although there is evidence that the two strategies work independently, I understand that the combination of the two strategies provides the best results overall.

There are at least two important reasons to favor the pulse approach. Insulin deactivates liver gluconeogenesis, that is, the production of glucose by the liver. When insulin is chronically suppressed for long periods, the liver begins to compensate for its lack by producing more glucose. As a result, your blood sugar starts rising even if you don't eat carbohydrates.

More importantly, in general many metabolic benefits associated with nutritional ketosis actually occur during the re-feeding phase. In the fasting phase, the removal of damaged cells and their contents occurs, but the real rejuvenation process takes place during re-feeding. In other words, the cells and tissues are rebuilt, and their healthy state is restored when the intake of net carbohydrates increases. (Rejuvenation during re-feeding is also one of the reasons why intermittent fasting has so many benefits, because you cycle hunger and abundance.)

How to Apply Cyclic Ketosis and Fasting?

- Take an intermittent fasting program – eat all meals (from breakfast to lunch, or from lunch to dinner) within an eight-hour time frame each day. Fast for the remaining 16 hours. If all of this is new to you and the idea of making changes in your diet and eating habits scares you too much, simply start by eating your usual meals during this time. Once it becomes a routine, continue implementing the ketogenic diet, and then making it cyclical. You can find comfort in knowing that once you reach the third step you can replenish some of your favorite healthy carbohydrates weekly.

- If you want to maximize the health benefits of fasting further, consider switching to regular five-day fasting on water alone. For example, I do it three or four times a year. To simplify this process, gradually reach a point where you fast for twenty hours a day and eat two meals in just four hours. After a month, fasting while consuming only water for five days will not be that difficult.

- Switch to a ketogenic diet until you generate measurable ketones – the three main stages are: limit the net carbohydrates (total carbohydrates without fiber) from 20 to 50 grams per day; replace the eliminated carbohydrates with healthy fats in order to obtain 50 to 85% of the daily caloric intake from fats and limit the protein to half a gram for every half kilo of lean body mass.

- Avoid all trans fats and polyunsaturated vegetable oils that are not fine. Adding these harmful fats can cause more damage than excess carbohydrates, so just because a food is "high in fat" doesn't mean you should eat it. Keep these portions of net carbohydrates, fats and proteins until you get into ketosis and your body burns fat as an energy source. To determine that you are ketotic, you can use the ketone test strips, checking that the ketones in your blood are in the range of 0.5 to 3.0 mmol/L. Remember that precision is important when it comes to portions of these nutrients. In fact, an excess of net carbohydrates will prevent ketosis as the body will first use any available glucose source, being a type of fuel that burns faster. Since it is practically impossible to determine the amount of fat accurately, net carbohydrates and proteins in all dishes, make sure you have some basic measuring and tracking tools at your fingertips.

- Once you have verified you are in ketosis, start cycling in and out of ketosis by replenishing high amounts of net carbohydrates once or twice a week. As a general recommendation, the amount of net carbohydrates triples during the days you fill up on carbohydrates.
- Remember that the body will again be able to effectively burn fat at any time after a couple of weeks or a few months.

As already mentioned, entering and exiting cyclically from nutritional ketosis will maximize biological benefits of regeneration and renewal, while at the same time minimizing potential negative sides of continuous ketosis. At this point, even if high or low carbohydrates are given once or twice a week, I would still advise you to be careful about what is healthy and what is not.

Do you want to get into keto and learn about how a low-carb diet can help with weight loss?

I wrote "Keto for Women Over 50" for people like you who need more than just information. You'll find an easy-to-follow 28-day meal plan too that is both practical and delicious, so there's no excuse not to give it a try!

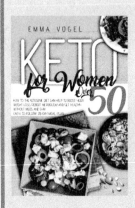

KETO FOR WOMEN OVER 50

How To The Ketogenic Diet Can Help To Boost Your Weight Loss, Reboot Metabolism And Get Healthy Without Meds And Gym

by Emma Vogel

US: https://www.amazon.com/dp/B08XLLDXHD

UK: https://www.amazon.co.uk/dp/B08XLLDXHD

CA: https://www.amazon.ca/dp/B08XLLDXHD

AU: https://www.amazon.com.au/dp/B08XLLDXHD

CHAPTER 5
BENEFITS

Improved Mental Concentration and Clarity

Fasting has incredible benefits for the healthy function of the brain. The most known benefit stems from the activation of autophagy, which is a cell cleansing process. Note that fasting has anti-seizure effects.

Longevity

This is the area in which we have had the highest amount of success. There is no doubt in the fact that the human race is living far much longer than what it used to live a few hundred years back. Just a century ago, the average lifespan of a human being at birth was less than half of what it is today. Women have been even luckier in terms of longer lifespan as studies show that on average, women live up to five years longer than men. In the US, the average life expectancy of a woman at the time of birth is 81.1 years, while the same for men is just 76.1 years.

Although we all want to live a long life and always think of it as a blessing, we all know that a long life in poor health is more of a curse than a blessing. It makes life dependent and miserable.

The second most desirable ingredient that can give a greater meaning to longevity is youthfulness.

Improvement in Hormone Profile

There are plenty of people who avoid intermittent fasting as they feel it will cause their fitness levels to deteriorate. This isn't necessarily the case for those people who do take part in intermittent fasting, as studies have shown that fasting does not negatively impact those who perform regular physical activities, especially if you cut down on your carbs as you fast and are in a ketosis state. Studies have shown that physical training while fasting can lead to higher metabolic adaptations.

Reduces Inflammation

Intermittent fasting promotes autophagy, a process in which the body destroys its old or damaged cells. Killing off old cells may sound like a terrible notion. However, it can be seen as a way of removing old and unwanted dirt from your body. It's a simple method for the body to clean and repair itself. Old and damaged cells can create inflammation. Because intermittent fasting stimulates autophagy, then it is possible to reduce inflammation in your body while fasting.

Polycystic Ovarian Syndrome and Intermittent Fasting

Polycystic ovaries are a fairly common disease in women. This disease causes a hormone shift and can have any undesirable effects on women. Many women struggle with weight gain and difficulty losing weight as a side effect of the disease.

While there are not very many studies about how intermittent fasting affects the disease, there is evidence that combining intermittent fasting with a keto diet significantly helped to regulate the hormones and made weight loss possible for polycystic ovarian syndrome patients. There does seem to be some potential hope with using intermittent fasting to help treat and maintain diseases like polycystic ovarian syndrome and other hormonal disorders. Time and additional research will tell us if intermittent fasting has a future in helping with this disease.

Lower the Risk of Diabetes

The most common health problem that plagues humanity these days, apart from obesity, is diabetes. High blood sugar leads to insulin resistance in the body.

Intermittent fasting helps to reduce blood sugar and therefore helps reduce insulin resistance in the body. When your body becomes resistant to insulin, it leads to an increase in the blood sugar level and the vicious cycle goes on and on. If you opt for this diet, you can successfully reverse this condition.

Improve Muscle Health

Many people get excited about the temporary weight reduction they experience when trying the crash diet. That is until they stop losing weight and eventually give up on a diet. But, most of the weight loss people achieve on these diets is not fat loss but water weight and muscle weight. Muscle weighs more than fat, so even a small amount of muscle loss can make a big difference on the scale.

As crash diets promote malnutrition, it naturally leads to

muscle loss, which negatively affects your health and strength as you age. After all, your muscles are in much more than your arms. They are surrounding your entire body, and even your heart is a muscle! As you lose muscle, your health and energy will be dramatically affected, and it is essential to regain this as you age if you want to improve your health.

Thankfully, studies have found that when compared to dieting, intermittent fasting not only leads to more weight loss than dieting, but it also causes much less muscle loss. This means your muscles will become much healthier, especially if you actively work out while you practice fasting.

Boosted Energy

The mitochondria, which are within our mitochondrial cells, are the powerhouse of the cell. It is the mitochondria that allow us to use a variety of fuel sources from the food we eat as fuel, as well as ketones. While other cells in the body may only be able to utilize one or two fuel types for energy, the mitochondria are incredibly versatile to be able to use all kinds of fuel. When you fast for longer periods (or are on a low-carb/ketogenic diet), your body begins to produce ketones, which are then used to cross the blood-brain barrier and fuel the brain in the absence of glucose. But that is not all. When you are in this fasted state of ketosis, the body will also increase the number of mitochondrial cells within your body, replacing non-mitochondrial cells with mitochondrial cells, allowing for more of your cells to be fueled by any fuel source.

Since the mitochondria fuel ninety percent of the human body, by increasing the number of these cells, you can naturally increase your energy. Not only will your physical energy increase, but your mental functioning and energy will, as well. This is great news for many people who lose energy as they age.

Lessen Oxidative Stress

Toxins cause oxidative stress. We can develop these toxins when we breathe in poor quality air, don't sleep well, eat poor quality food, apply damaging substances to our skin, and much more. We even develop this oxidative stress when our cells convert fuel to energy, meaning that even if we live in a clean environment, sleep perfectly, and only eat organic food, we would still develop oxidative stress, thereby causing damage to our cells. As our cells develop this damage from oxidative stress, we slowly lose our health and energy, producing an increased risk of disease. However, studies have shown that intermittent fasting not only increases the rate our cells develop oxidative stress, but it also increases our body's natural antioxidants to fight against this damage directly.

Improve Mental Well-Being

Poor mental health is becoming more common than ever, with over forty million Americans suffering from one form of mental illness or another, and many others struggling with short-term depression and anxiety. One of the most common causes of disability in middle-aged Americans (as well as those who are young) is chronic severe depression. Yet, a majority of these people never seek professional help.

While I urge you always to seek professional help for your mental health, you can also practice intermittent fasting. Studies have found that with short-term fasting, people can significantly improve their everyday mood, tranquility, alertness, and even the feeling of euphoria. Not only that but also the symptoms of severe depression can be improved with fasting.

Heart's Health

Heart disease is the most significant killer in the world. Several risk factors increase the chance of heart disease. Intermittent fasting helps reduce risk factors like blood pressure, high cholesterol, inflammatory markers, blood sugar and blood triglycerides. When you can control these risk factors, you reduce the chance of suffering from cardiovascular disease. However, once again, a lot of research in this field is based on animal studies.

Cellular Repair

Autophagy is the process of waste removal in the body, and intermittent fasting helps to kick-start this process. The body breaks down and metabolizes broken, as well as dysfunctional, proteins. An increase in autophagy protects you from several degenerative diseases like cancer and Alzheimer's.

All these benefits help to increase your lifespan and help

you lead a healthier life. Not only will you lose weight, but you can also improve your overall health just by following the intermittent fasting method.

Boosts Your Immune System

As a result of the many benefits that you gain from intermittent fasting, you also get to look forward to having an improved immune system. This is from the combination of reduced physical stress, increased cellular reparation abilities, weight loss, and other benefits that you gain from intermittent fasting.

Improved Sex Drive

Lower levels of production in both estrogen and testosterone may lead to a decreased sex drive. As such, it is not a psychological or physiological issue, but it is a hormonal matter.

So, when you engage in intermittent fasting, your brain will regain its balance and begin to produce the right levels of all hormones. So, in addition to improving your cognitive ability, restricting the production of cortisol, and boosting your mood through increased production of endorphins and dopamine, your body will also regulate the production of estrogen and testosterone which could potentially lead to a healthier sex drive.

Cellular Repair

Autophagy is the process of waste removal in the body, and intermittent fasting helps to kick-start this process. The body breaks down and metabolizes broken, as well as dysfunctional, proteins. An increase in autophagy protects you from several degenerative diseases like cancer and Alzheimer's.

All these benefits help to increase your lifespan and help you lead a healthier life. Not only will you lose weight, but you can also improve your overall health just by following the intermittent fasting method.

CHAPTER 6
SUCCESS STORIES

Every day, we are seeing an increase in the use of intermittent fasting to help women over 50 achieve a healthier body and mind. The results for many can be just as dramatic as the results of popular dieting plans like the 5:2.

Women report enjoying higher energy levels, weight loss, and anti-aging benefits of the program. They might have restricted their eating window, but are still munching on scrumptious foods throughout the day while seeing results of losing 2 to 4lbs a week.

Melanie, 54 years old, Dallas Texas.

"I'm always looking for ways to improve my health. I'm 54 years old and I used to weigh 168lbs. And I am the first to admit that I am no expert on health, diet, or anything related to that. I also want to do some experimentation and find out what my body can and can't handle. I had a friend (let's call her Joanne) who lost 22lbs, but still, her diet was not so bad. She liked to eat fish once every two days and some kind of meat or other vegetarian foods. I asked her how was she able to lose 10 kilos in three months, and she said, 'Intermittent fasting!'

I got hooked on the idea, but I got scared of the fact of whether I'd drop it just like the other diet trends I had tried in the past. I talked to Joanne on how to get started, and she told me to take it slow and easy. I would choose my eating window if I couldn't get past the stricter timetables. Joanne told me she had a hard time adjusting at first. She started with the 16:8 intermittent fasting timetable. I would like to do the same.

I have to clear out my health conditions to my doctor before joining Joanne. Other than the fact I'm asthmatic, there's nothing else to worry about. Fast forward, I started intermittent fasting at a 16:8 eating window.

I will often start to experiment with my meal plan to have an idea of what to expect from the coming week. I've learned that if I begin to plan my food the week before, I often eat less during the diet and don't experience the hunger that I do when I try to

Emma Vogel

prepare for it a few days beforehand.

After a period of familiarization, I try to do some internet research and think about what I expect to eat and the impact it will have on my energy levels and mood. I lost about 21lbs for four months! It was hard and slower than some women, but, I'm glad I was able to make that change. I jogged around the neighborhood and that helped a lot in burning more calories than expected."

Connie, 51 years old, Seattle, Washington.

"When it comes to diet, fads come and go. So, when I got an email recently from someone saying she's done "losing weight by eating a low-carb diet," I thought she was probably exaggerating for effect. I agreed with her that it can be a good strategy because eating fewer carbs makes you lose weight. And lots of people on the keto diet think it has helped them lose weight and feel better. But, I asked myself whether it'll work for me. I know I can be lazy to pick up a diet and continue working with it. In 2016, I had to make a lifestyle change due to a kidney condition. As a result, I was placed on kidney dialysis three times. So, with the support of my husband, I knew I had to make some changes in my diet and my lifestyle to maintain my health.

I chose intermittent fasting because my doctor 'Okayed' with it. I was motivated by the fact that even if I was not restricting my diet the weight would come off slowly but surely. My 30-day intermittent fasting was successful.

I ate a lot of salad without any dressing, that's for sure. That was done in two weeks and I have lost 10 pounds so far. My husband went along with it, because he felt good about his health, too. Besides, I do need a partner in this journey as we got into a better shape ourselves."

Patty, 52 years old, Tampa, Florida.

My husband and I started doing intermittent fasting together in 2018. You know, 'Hey, let's do it together,' and then we started doing it for longer periods. We did it once in 2014, but it wasn't very successful for both of us. And then one day in March 2018, we were both like, 'Okay, we're going to commit to this.'

We were losing about 3lbs per week! We eat breakfast, lunch, and dinner with occasional snacks and desserts.

And then, I quit my job, so I could just focus on the diet and lose weight. My husband followed suit. So, we decided to just focus on the diet and work on our bodies at home together. And as long as we stick to that, it just worked.

And, you know, I felt great. I felt happy. I was losing weight. It was something that we could do together, and it wasn't that difficult of a diet. I think it's important for us to let people know that you don't have to do something hard to succeed on it.

I'm telling people about it because, if you feel like you want to do it, you could try it with your significant other, with your friend, with anybody.

We have friends who do intermittent fasting with each other, so you can do it with your friends. I've also seen people do it with their husbands and wives.

This is a nice way to help lose weight—to have a support network. So, we got pretty far. We got to the point where we were both able to give up alcohol and coffee, and we weren't hungry anymore in the mornings. So we just wanted to share our story because we felt empowered. And we felt like we could do anything.

Sarah, 56 years old, Philadelphia, Pennsylvania.

At 50 years old, I was a Creative Marketing Senior weighing 174lbs. I was 5ft. 6in. tall and had a potbelly, and bulging saggy breasts. I felt frustrated, unattractive, and unhealthy in the workplace, especially around new and younger hires.

In October of 2015, my husband and I decided to head back to Philly to live near my parents. I've quit my job and was busy setting up my new events and wedding business. From there, I joined a gym and started training to start a new lifestyle.

But, when I went to the gym after work, I was super self-conscious, embarrassed, and ashamed of myself. I just simply wanted to hide in the comforts of my own home. I stopped exercising that's for sure.

I looked through the mirror after every workout session, only to discover that none made me feel great for weeks afterward.

Just like other people, I was Googling how to lose weight and I've read about intermittent fasting. I decided to follow that program because I could do it at home without getting embarrassed about exercising to lose weight. I didn't even share this with my husband for two months until he saw the changes in me!

When I told him I was fasting, he was supportive of me. He always knew about my insecurities. While he didn't exactly join me on my new diet plan, he went along eating what's in the fridge — healthy foods. So, I did it for about five months, and I would have to make myself wake up at 5 AM or 6 AM to eat. It was hard. It was hard. So I would suggest that if you're willing to commit, that you stick with it for a long time.

I lost about 26lbs in five months. I finally got the courage to exercise by the half of the second month with my husband. That made me losing weight done faster.

Right now in my 50s, I'm a happy events planner ready to face clients and tackle the world.

Emma Vogel

Nina, 51, Denver, Colorado.

After a horrible accident eight years ago, I'd like to think that I've let go of myself to any food that I want because I felt like I deserved it. From there, I grew heavy. Not to mention, my accident made it difficult to exercise, especially with my left arm.

When I had a medical checkup on my acid reflux, my doctor said that I should lose some weight to ease my digestive tract from heartburn. She recommended me to start walking or jogging and cutting back carbs.

For someone who does not exercise or listen to fad diets, of course, I'll be confused. 'How do I begin to do that?' I've searched online and tried various slimming pills for an easy way out.

However, I had kidney pains from swallowing them every day. I even burped hard and smelly back then. Fortunately, the pain didn't come out as severe as it is. I chugged a lot of water to ease the pain. It did.

When a cousin told me about intermittent fasting, I bluffed it off. If I did not have the discipline to exercise or eat properly before, how would I ever follow the fasting method successfully? I was scared. So, I asked for help from my doctor about the regimen.

For me not to break off the cycle of my fast, I downloaded an app in iOS to track my eating window.

Eating and prepping food was a little problem for me. It was all about the habit, mindset, and continuity. Fast forward to five months, my body weight dropped around 57lbs.

The experience was liberating. The only time food entered my diet was during periods of extreme hunger. But I ate my favorite food like crazy for days straight, while consuming enough energy from fish, avocados, eggs, etc.

Some may be skeptical as this will take you too far into what is known among scientists as 'starvation.' I was skeptical too.

But, it worked for me. My body adjusted and my stomach grew accustomed to hunger. So, here's what I'm going to say: It gets difficult, but, it gets better.

CHAPTER 7
5 BEST METHODS OF INTERMITTENT FASTING FOR WOMEN OVER 50

Since the introduction of intermittent fasting, several different variations of this diet have become available for people to follow. Each of these variations has unique benefits that can be gained, as well as considerations for you to think about. They are designed to support you with different goals and assist you in maintaining your best levels of health. While there are practically countless adaptations of the intermittent fasting diet out there, we are going to focus on just five in this chapter. Each of these diets adjusts the levels of fasting that you will experience on either a daily or weekly basis. Some will require more fasting than others, whereas some offer more eating time. If you decide after some trial and error that the one you have chosen does not fit your needs or feels too challenging for you to maintain, consider trying a different adaptation. However, make sure that you give each one at least a few weeks of effort to ensure that the challenges you are facing are not simply you are getting used to your new diet. Once you have found the one that works for you, simply maintain it, and continue receiving all of the great benefits from it!

Time-Restricted Eating (16:8 Method)

The 16:8 fasting diet is similar to the 12-hour fast except that it requires a slightly longer fasting window. This fasting diet can be a little more challenging for some people to adapt to as it requires 16 hours of fasting and only 8 hours of eating. This means that in 8 hours you need to consume any meals and snacks that you want to for the day.

Despite being more intense, the 16:8 diet is still typically an easy one to adjust to. With some minor adjustments to your daily schedule, you can easily accommodate to the longer fasting window. Typically, most people who do the 16:8 diet simply cut out their regular breakfast meal and just focus on lunch and dinner instead. This makes it quite a simple adjustment once you get used to skipping breakfast. The most common way of eating in alignment with this fast is to stop eating at 8 PM each day and then eat again at noon the next day. This is typically the easiest way to accommodate for the 16 hours of fasting. However, you can also choose to stop eating after dinner and eat an earlier lunch the next day. How you choose to adjust the fasting window is not nearly as important as making sure that you get the full 16 hours of fasting in each day.

For some people, the 16:8 diet may still be quite similar to how they already eat. For both the 12-hour fast and the 16:8 diet, many people find that they instinctively eat this way, to begin with. However, being stricter about not eating during that fasting window can support you in seeing greater health benefits from your dietary habits. The 16:8 fasting diet is the level of intermittent fasting where many of the most optimal benefits are truly gained. Studies have shown that this variation of the diet is optimal for anyone who is looking to protect against obesity, inflammation, diabetes, and liver disease. These benefits can all be gained even if you continue to consume the same number of calories per day, simply in a shorter window of time. The primary beneficial health factor here is the longer fasting, not the number of calories consumed.

The Twice-a-Week (5:2 method)

The original diet to ever be shared and popularized when it came to intermittent fasting was the 5:2 fasting diet. This is a weekly diet, not a daily diet like the previous two we discussed. For the 5:2 fasting diet, you eat as you normally would five days a week and then significantly reduce your calorie intake for two days a week. This ratio is said to support you in gaining all of the benefits of intermittent fasting with relatively little interruption to your regular eating habits.

For the two days that you are fasting, you are still allowed to have a small amount of calorie intake. Typically, men will consume about 600 calories per day and women will consume about 500 calories per day. This gives you enough to refrain from starving, but without interrupting your fast too much.

The most common way to complete the 5:2 diet is to distribute the days throughout the week. Rather than fasting two days in a row, people will fast on one day, eat for three, fast on one day, and eat for two. This ensures that you do not feel as though you are going too long between meals. That way, you maintain your hunger satisfied and your diet remains sustainable.

For the 5:2 diet, a study was done that showed that more than 100 women who were either overweight or obese lost the same amount of weight using this eating method as they did when restricting calories. However, restricting calories is typically more intense and harder to maintain over time. Many people who restrict calories on a continued basis find themselves struggling to maintain the restriction over time. Furthermore, any time they stop restricting their calories they see more weight gain which can lead to continuous changes in weight. This is not only upsetting to the person dieting but can also be stressful and unhealthy to their body.

Alternating Day Fasting

Alternating which day you fast on is a common variation of the intermittent fasting diet. It also happens to have many of its own unique adaptations. Typically, the one you choose is based on what feels best for you and supports you in getting the best results. Some people choose to completely avoid any solid foods on their fasting days whereas others will eat up to

500 calories on their fasting days. On days where the individual eats normally, they can eat as much as they want. This is a more intense version of the intermittent fasting diet, and it may take more work to acclimate your body to this dieting habit so that you can maintain it properly. You may also prefer to start with eating up to 500 calories and then reduce to having no solids on your fasting days, or you might just stay with 500 calorie days. For this variation of the diet, the best way to find what works is to play around a bit and see what feels best for you.

Studies have shown that alternating fasting days is effective in supporting individuals with their heart health. It is also an incredible variation for people who want to lose weight. One study that was conducted found that the average person lost about 11 pounds over a 12-week period using this diet. Because of how extreme this fasting diet can be, it is not ideal for anyone who has never fasted before. Even if you have naturally fasted for fairly extended periods of time, you should first work towards intentionally sustaining a more relaxed variation of the intermittent fasting diet before moving to alternating days. You should also avoid this fasting style if you are dealing with certain medical conditions as it can have a negative impact on you. If you are considering the alternating day's diet for intermittent fasting, be sure to let your doctor know your specific plans. This can help them determine what would be the right decision for you to make so that you don't face any adverse health repercussions.

Eat Stop Eat (24-Hour Fast)

Similar to the 5:2 fast is the 24-hour weekly fast. This variation of the diet allows people to consume food normally six days per week, and then completely fast for 24 hours. During this 24-hour window, absolutely no food should be consumed. Individuals are also encouraged to avoid drinking any drinks that may be too high in calories, such as whole milk lattés or smoothies.

This variation of the diet is often called the "eat-stop-eat" diet because it only requires one day of true change on a weekly basis. Otherwise, you can eat whatever you want and however, you want. For those who are seeking to incorporate weekly dieting into their eating plans, the 24-hour weekly fast is a great place to start. This is a relatively relaxed place to start. For some people, it may offer plenty enough benefits to make it a good place to stay, too. For others, they may prefer to adjust to the 5:2 diet after they get used to it so that they can see greater results from their efforts.

It is important to be cautious of how the 24-hour weekly fast impacts you. While some people find great success with this, other people find that one single day per week is not frequently enough, so their body never fully acclimates. As a result, they end up experiencing headaches, fatigue, or even irritability during their fasting day. For most, these symptoms outweigh the benefits that they gain, which results in them not maintaining the 24-hour fasting cycle. If you still want to give this eating pattern a try, you may benefit from first using the 16:8 fasting method before adjusting to test out the 24-hour weekly fasting. This can support your body with getting used to the changes.

Spontaneous Meal Skipping

Meal skipping is an extremely flexible form of intermittent fasting that can provide all of the benefits of intermittent fasting but with less of the strict scheduling. If you are not someone who has a typical schedule or who feels as though a more strict variation of the intermittent fasting diet will serve you, meal skipping is a viable alternative.

Many people who choose to use meal skipping find it to be a great way to listen to their bodies and follow their basic instincts. If they are not hungry, they simply don't eat that meal. Instead, they wait for the next one. Meal skipping can also be helpful for people who have time constraints and who may not always be able to get in a certain meal of the day.

It is important to realize that with meal skipping, you may not always be maintaining a 10-16-hour window of fasting. As a result, you may not get every benefit that comes from other fasting diets. However, this may be a great solution for people who want an intermittent fasting diet that feels more natural to them. It may also be a great idea for those who are looking to begin listening to their body more so that they can adjust to a more intense variation of the diet with greater ease. In other words, it can be a great transitional diet for you if you are not ready to jump into one of the other fasting diets just yet.

PART 2: THE 14-DAY PROGRAM

CHAPTER 8
How to Start

"Beginning is the hardest but is worth it at the end," unknown.

With the spirit of the above quote in mind, let's begin a step-by-step guide on exactly how to fast intermittently.

Get Clear on Your Goals

Having clear goals can take you far in life generally, but don't underestimate the importance of defining your objectives before you begin an IF regimen. For me, it was losing the excess weight I had put on during and after pregnancy (this consequently solved a bunch of other health issues for me), improving metabolic health as well as achieving mental sharpness and focus. Broadly speaking, I wanted to experience overall better health for my own sake, and most importantly, my baby's. However, my research indicated that I needed to define exactly what I wanted out of IF in order to reap its full benefits.

And let me explain why this is the case.

Defining your goals when it comes to IF is critical for a number of reasons. First and foremost, it allows you to pick the most suitable IF method that will effectively take you closer to what you want. For instance, the Alternate-Day IF method is more fitting for those aiming to lose weight, while the 16:8 method is more of a healthy lifestyle change. While weight loss is one of the most popular reasons people embark on an IF journey, you might have your own reasons for giving IF a chance. Find out what you want out of the diet and then move to the step below.

Choose Your Method

Now that you know exactly what you're seeking from IF, the next step involves picking a suitable IF method that will help you achieve your goals. In addition to your specific goals regarding IF, there are other factors that also go into choosing an IF method that would yield the most benefits for you. These include the length of time you want to fast for, your daily routine, what field you work in, what a typical workday looks like for you, and the specific climatic conditions prevailing in your part of the world, and how often you dine out with friends and family — to name a few.

Once you have chosen an IF method, though, remember that you're not stuck with it forever. It is completely possible to transition from one type of IF to another if you find that your current regimen isn't working for you or if you think you've mastered the moderate forms of IF (think of the 16:8 method) and want to go pro and explore some relatively challenging routes such as the alternate-day fasting. Besides, it is advisable for a person to give at least one month's serious go to any particular IF method before quitting or switching it up for good.

Identify Your Calorie Needs

Now that you know what you want from IF and how you're going to approach it, the next step involves finding a way to figure out and manage your calories. This is important because if your top goal for IF is weight loss, then you need to consume fewer calories than you burn for energy, i.e., build a calorie-deficit. While IF is naturally designed to create a calorie deficit when you're fasting, this can be quickly turned into a surplus if you're not mindful of the calories you consume during your eating windows.

Some people practicing IF are usually the least concerned about counting and measuring the calories they consume. Although keeping track of one's calorie consumption is important to a certain extent (even while fasting intermittently), these folks are of the opinion that their calorie consumption is automatically taken care of as a direct result of fasting intermittently. While this may work out well for someone who doesn't suffer from (or is prone to) an eating disorder such as anorexia, orthorexia, and binge eating, it can be detrimental for individuals whose eating disorders may be triggered by IF. Keeping track of the number of calories you consume during IF is also important because even if certain methods of IF such as the Alternate-Day fasting do allow for calorie consumption during fasting days, there is a limit to how much of these calories one can consume. Again, this restriction is meant to facilitate the benefits of IF such as weight loss. Besides, there is a popular opinion that as long as you consume just under 50 calories in the morning, you will be considered to be in the fasting state. This can be critical for those practicing the 16:8 method by having an early dinner and delayed breakfast in an attempt to reach a 16-hour milestone with their fasting. Such people can drink plain water or have a cup of black coffee (no added sugar!) without the risk of breaking their fast in the mornings.

But, guess what, this also implies that you have to be mindful of the calories you consume in order to make sure that your IF regimen is not put to waste. All of this leads to one conclusion, whether you're fasting or feasting, you must keep an eye on your calorie consumption in order to achieve your goals with IF. At least in the beginning.

Nowadays, there are a variety of apps that can be used to track calorie intake. Some of the best ones include "MyFitnessPal" and "Lose It," which not only include a calorie counter but also boast a food diary and an exercise log.

As you get the hang of doing IF in any way or form that you think best suits you and your situation, the focus on calorie intake will usually wind up fading into the background as IF and your new eating habits get ingrained into your schedule. You will find that you do not need to track the calories as much because you know the approximate amounts which you consume on a daily basis. This is when the much-vaunted benefit of not needing to count calories comes back straight into play, with a vengeance! Because you have more practice and have already established a fair routine and habit of doing your IF lifestyle, your daily caloric intake is more or less at your fingertips. Consequently, you end up not having to pay too much attention to that, as you are able to carry on with your daily stuff without having to worry about the calorie count.

Conduct Meal Planning Without Overdoing It

And no. I'm not about to contradict myself here.

IF is quite liberating in the sense that it allows one to let go of the tedious job of meal planning all the time. And I'm not going back on my words here. This step is, in fact, pretty optional. You can choose to do it, or not. IF is not a practice meant to put restrictions on someone when it comes to what they eat. Nonetheless, we all know that a balanced and nutritious diet is critical for maintaining good health, regardless of whether or not you practice IF. One thing that must be understood is that restricting food for a certain number of hours does not justify consuming junk food when the eating window finally opens. Making unhealthy food choices when you finally sit down to eat in an IF regimen is not only detrimental for your overall health but will also put any and all of your efforts with regards to IF go to waste.

And you don't want that.

Therefore, it is recommended that you take some time out to (informally) plan what you will eat during say, the week ahead. This will not help you keep track of your calorie intake (and thereby lose and maintain weight consistently) but also ensure that you have everything you need to cook a healthy, nutritious and delicious meal on hand.

Because let's be honest, we are more susceptible to ordering takeaway food, and eating unhealthy snacks when prepping a healthy meal at home becomes difficult due to any reason. And frankly, if you find yourself eating loads of unhealthy food when you aren't fasting, you might as well not fast at all!

Emma Vogel

Begin Your IF Journey with the Pedal to the Metal

Once you have completed all of the steps above, you are now ready to begin your IF journey and see where it takes you.

Along with all of my very best wishes, here are a few things that I would like you to keep in mind while you're at it:

- Make the calories count in the beginning by keeping the nutritional value of any food you consume in insight.
- Practice moderation, both while fasting and feasting.
- Take IF as an opportunity to improve your eating habits and food choices. Fewer meals mean more time for preparing healthy food to dine on.
- IF isn't a one-size-fits-all approach, so keep experimenting to figure out what works best for you.

CHAPTER 9
MISTAKES TO AVOID

Making Lots of Changes within a Short Duration

It is natural to get too excited when you are about to start something new; you can't wait to have all the rewards that come with it, so you probably want to dive into it. However, you need to caution that trying to make lots of changes in a few weeks can prevent you from enjoying all the rewards you seek. Hence, you must start slowly and grow into it; an instance is adopting the 5:2 method where you eat only 500 calories all through the day twice a week and feed "normal" on the remaining five days. You may start by eating 500 calories once in the week and having regular meals for the remaining six days. After 2-3 weeks, you can add the second day, and from there, you can adopt other methods with more extended fasting periods.

Not Monitoring Your Liquid Intake

It is essential to know that your fasting state can come to an end not only when you eat, but also when you drink the liquids, you are not supposed to. Some liquids will break your fast and deny you the fast benefits, even if they are calorie or fat-free. Diet sodas and sweeteners are some of the liquids you should stay away from; sweetener can cause a spike in your insulin levels. The main liquid you are permitted to take while doing intermittent fasting is water. Moderate black coffee is also allowed. Adding lemon to your water or sugar to the coffee will also nullify your fast.

Not Drinking Adequate Water

It is recommended to drink a lot of water while engaging in intermittent fasting. If you refuse to drink enough water while fasting, it can make you dehydrated and very thirsty, and it is possible to confuse thirst for hunger.

The International Food Information has already stated that 20% of the water the body uses comes from the foods we feed on. At the same time, since you are intermittent fasting, your food intake will be limited; hence, you need to drink 20% more water than usual to make up for the foods.

Feeding on Unhealthy Foods

Intermittent fasting is not a diet plan; hence, it doesn't prevent you from eating your food choice. The freedom of having the luxury to eat any meal has made a lot of people fall into a "trap" as they feed on junks or breaking their fast with fast food. Desist from the habit of feeding on unhealthy meals with the mindset that your fasts would cover up for you.

To enjoy all the health benefits of intermittent fasting, it is essential to feed on healthy foods. When you visit the grocery store, buy foods rich in protein, calcium, and B-12.

Overeating When You Break Your Fast

This is a prevalent mistake most beginners of intermittent fasting make. Even those who practice intermittent fasting in the past and claim it doesn't work mostly do this. If you eat lots of calorie-filled meals when you break your fast and are trying to lose weight, you probably might not be able to achieve your aim.

To avoid overeating, you should feed on large quantities of healthy foods during your eating period. This food should be made up of fresh vegetables and healthy salads. You should also have your meal prepared before your fasting period ends; this will prevent you from eating just anything when your fasting period elapses.

Sticking with the Wrong Plan

There are several plans for intermittent fasting. It is essential to study each of these plans and adopt one that can easily be integrated into your daily routine. If your work requires you to leave home very early in the morning to engage in strenuous jobs, the fasting plan whereby you won't eat from 8 pm until after 12 pm the following day will be a wrong plan for you as this will not augur well with your job.

It is essential to know that the intermittent fasting plan that works for someone else might not work for you. Hence, you can experiment with the various methods available and study each of them as it applies to you to see the one that gives you the best result.

CHAPTER 10
EXERCISE TO DO WITH INTERMITTENT FASTING DIET

Women over fifty have a hard time taking care of their bodies if they are not active. Our body is not healthy if it is subjected to a sedimentary lifestyle for too long. There are several reasons for this. Some of the most active women I have seen in their fifties moved a lot around their bodies. They exercised their bodies, keeping fit easily even as they aged. There were also cases of women who were only forty-five years old, but had the problems of women sixty-five years older. I expected as much as seeing their sedimentary lifestyle.

Exercise makes a big difference. When you move through your body, you automatically push it to regulate its functions, with a good performance. The body needs exercise just as our functions must work well. Exercise is what makes the difference the most. It is that healthy habit that decides whether you will automatically have a thirty-year-old body while staying fifty or have a sixty-five-year-old body while still being forty. Generally, there are two types of females. The first type of women includes those women who have been active in their youth. When they were in their twenties or even thirty, they moved quite a bit. Yoga, jogging, and aerobics are something they know. Naturally, they are also women who can do intermittent fasting better. Even if you are a woman in your fifties, you will stay much fitter if you exercised in your prime.There is another type of female that has led to a sedimentary lifestyle. These women are often inactive, with no interest in exercise or physical activity. Often, the busy routine, coupled with the field of work, makes this possible.I can give you good news. Women who haven't exercised in their twenties or even thirties can still reap the benefits of exercise. As you do intermittent fasting, you will find that your bodies are more mobile than before, and you can easily do things you didn't think were possible.

Even if you were a woman who had led a life of physical inactivity, you still have a chance. Intermittent fasting naturally lowers cholesterol, leading to a free and active body. For women who have been quite active before and still exercise a great deal, I would suggest cutting back a bit. Intermittent fasting combined with exercise is a powerful combination for losing weight and lowering cholesterol. However, you must avoid exhaustion. I will give a list of the best exercises that are suitable for women over fifty. You can choose a suitable time for these exercises, such as in the morning or in the evening. Make sure you don't strain your body too much. Your body is your temple and the more you take care of it, the more it will take care of you.

Walking/Jogging

This exercise is for the females who have led an inactive lifestyle. You can start with a thirty-minute walk in the park or even your home. Gradually increase it to forty-five minutes if possible. Walking is an amazing exercise if practiced daily. It is also the most basic form of exercise, leading females into a sense of activity. Interestingly, it is also preferred by women who were once very active but now have gone inactive physically.

The best thing about walking is that it can be done on your street or even rooftop. An advanced form of walking is jogging. You can try it out in the park. When you start walking and then gradually move towards jogging, there are a lot of benefits you

Emma Vogel

will reap. Not only will your physical body be more active, but your mental health will also benefit from it.

Light Aerobics

Don't have much time? Or maybe it is not possible to cross the street or the park? Light aerobics may be what you need. You can start with light aerobics or low-impact aerobics. There are many YouTube videos available online. You can start from there. You will only have to do this for 20 minutes a day, three to four days a week. The great thing about aerobics is that it easily provides an incredible exercise in no time.

It does not require any equipment. All you need is a laptop to watch videos on them and space like a room. Don't put too much pressure on your body. The video fellows are experts. You just have to do the exercise and move your body.

Stretching/Yoga

Stretching exercises are naturally the best. You can easily do adult yoga every day. The best results are obtained when combined with light aerobics or walking. Yoga or stretching exercises have immense benefits. They relieve joint pain, give bones strength and flexibility, and increase their immunity. Stretching exercises also allow your body to be more flexible and strong. Other than that, your mind will relax while your body does the stretch. Yoga poses for adult women are readily available online. The same rule applies here with light aerobics as well. You will have to take it easy. Just stretch your body until you feel slight discomfort. Don't push too hard.

A yoga routine is readily available. If you are someone who hasn't exercised in years, then yoga is for you too. Naturally, the best duo I've seen in some women was doing gentle yoga in the morning and combining it with light aerobics or walking at night. In case you do intermittent fasting, even simple yoga might be enough.

Balance

There are plenty of light exercises that focus on improving your balance. Naturally, some poses of yoga also focus on balance. It is somewhat a crucial part of your health. You should focus on it quite often.

CHAPTER 11
Tips for Maintaining Intermittent Fasting

Drinking Water and Organic Juices

Many scientific studies have indicated that intermittent fasting is beneficial and has many advantages which primarily benefit the brain and other organs in our bodies. Intermittent fasting induces many metabolic changes in our bodies. One of the most important is that it drops blood sugar levels to manageable limits and cuts down on fat. The drop in insulin levels encourages the burning of accumulated fat. When the stomach realizes that there is no food coming in, it would inform the brain, which conveys to all the accumulated fat to burn up and provide the energy that the body needs to function. In such a situation, you should avoid drinks that contain "Lucine" which is an enzyme that helps in the synthesis of protein, which would send the wrong signals to the brain. The brain would react and then send around the wrong signals around your body and prevent the breakdown or synthesis of fat which is protein to provide the body's energy. Preventing the synthesis of protein would result in you not losing weight which would be one of the main reasons to practice intermittent fasting in the first place. It is as simple as that. That is why intermittent fasting has become very popular worldwide, and many are practicing it very regularly. It is just one aspect of the benefit of intermittent fasting.

There are many more all happening within your body as the monotonousness of the metabolic system is disturbed when the regular food intake is denied. The body is accustomed to the regular three meals or more a day and the system works with the excess fats being deposited all over the body, sugar levels allowed to increase without any control and other regulars like the uncontrolled intake of sweetened drinks and different types of food that are generally detrimental to our bodies being consumed. If stopped during intermittent fasting, all these would give a wake up call to our bodies and then the body has to do with whatever it has stored to keep the energy flowing to ensure that the system works at an optimum level. Just because you did not consume a meal or two in intermittent times the body is not ready to shut down and let you die, it would ensure that you stay alive. While intermittent fasting may be useful for the body and mind, there are certain precautions. Anyone who is on a fast should avoid creating other problems because of the brief.

As you could consume liquids, it would be wise to know what would be acceptable and what could do you more harm than good or even worse, to make you seriously ill. Hence, it would help if you took serious note of what you would consume in liquids when you are intermittent fasting. Of course, you would not partake of any solid form meals because you are on a fast. Still, there would not be any restrictions to consume water and other organic juices during that period, but "what" is the big question.

There is a wide variety of organic juices that you could consume but know what they constitute before you gulp it down your throat would be prudent. Water is acceptable as you would need to be well hydrated throughout your fast. There should not be any reason for the body to be wanting in water because water is required to ensure that the blood that circulates the body has ample water to lubricate. Water is essential because it ensures that all the nutrients are carried around the body and is adequately supplied to all the organs whilst also taking away the waste from our bodies to be disposed of. Hence water should be taken in moderate quantities to ensure that the above processes are not hindered which could have adverse reactions in the body.

The next question that would arise is how good are the different organic juice's and just to name a few, apple, orange, carrot, tomatoes, vegetable, and coconut water. The critical aspect here would be the quantity of sugar that would consist of what it would do inside your body because sugar has to be controlled during intermittent fasting. When you are on an intermittent fast, the body is denied sugar and to counter this. The body produces more insulin to ensure that the sugar within is managed adequately, which controls the "blood sugar" levels. When blood sugar levels are controlled, insulin is maintained at optimum levels and neither increased nor reduced.

It is one crucial aspect that is right for your health when on an intermittent fast. You would disturb this equilibrium between "blood sugar" levels and insulin production when you consume excess quantities of high sugar-based organic juices.

High on the list to be avoided, is

- Apple juice which has 10 grams of sugar in 100 grams of fluid, hence should be avoided at all costs
- Orange juice with 8.9 grams of sugar in 100 grams of juice trails a close second, then comes
- Carrot juice which has 3.9 grams of sugar in 100 grams of liquid, next is
- Tomatoes which is also high in sugar with 3.6 grams of it in 100 grams of juice,
- Vegetable juice, which has 2.1 grams of sugar in 100 grams of liquid, would depend on the vegetables you choose. The "new kid in the block" which is taking the world by storm for all the good things it has to offer and becoming very popular indeed is
- Coconut water has one of the lowest quantities of sugar in 100 grams of water with only 2.6 grams of it just trailing behind vegetable juice.

Hence it is imperative that if you are on an intermittent fast and need to derive all the benefits from it, you should be prudent in what you consume during and after the short.

CHAPTER 12
WHAT TO EAT TO AVOID HUNGRY PAINS

Water

This is definitely the most important element to consume when you take up the intermittent fast. Water can act as an elixir when it comes to losing weight. You must keep your body hydrated and ensure that all the toxins are dissolved and eliminated. All your organs need water to remain fresh and healthy; right from your liver to gut, to digestive tract, water helps to keep these organs working smoothly. Drink at least 8 to 10 glasses of water a day and focus more on the fasting period. It is obvious that it will get a little monotonous and so, a good idea is to consume fruit-infused water. This refers to water that has fruit and herbs infused into it. Fill up a jar with water and toss in fruit and herbs such as oranges, lemons, mint leaves, and a dash of cinnamon. Consume this every few hours. Remember that the intermittent fast can be quite taxing at times and lead to side effects such as headaches and nausea. In such a case, only water can help you out and put an end to these.

Fish

Fish can be considered a miracle food as it can greatly help with weight loss. According to dietary guidelines, it is important for people to consume at least 6 to 8 ounces of fish every week. Fish contains a lot of nutrients. It is rich in fats and proteins.

It is also rich in vitamin D. This means you do not have to worry about denying your body these nutrients by taking on the fast. You do not have to reach for supplements if you can consume fish regularly. Fish is also rich in DHA, which helps in brain development. You will see that your mind is fresher and you are able to think well. Your productivity will increase and stress will be curbed.

Avocado

You might wonder why avocado is on this list considering it is one of the fattiest foods out there. However, you must understand that the fasting phase can take a toll on your body and so you must consume foods that can keep you going. Avocado is rich in monounsaturated fat, which is great for those who tend to get hungry quite fast. It keeps you feeling full for longer. You will not find yourself reaching out to eat a snack. Avocado is quite versatile and can be added to your breakfast or lunch menu.

Those who tend to include it in their breakfast menu are generally able to go without food for longer periods without complaining about hunger.

Leafy Greens

If there is one type of vegetable that we remember being told to consume by our parents then it has to be leafy green vegetables. As we know, leafy green vegetables are loaded with multiple nutrients that are great for your body. These include kale, broccoli, lettuce, etc. These are loaded with fiber. Fiber, as you know, keeps your body going when you suffer from digestive issues such as constipation. You are sure to go through it when you adopt the intermittent fast. In such a case, it becomes that much more important to consume these vegetables to keep your stomach in good shape. Fiber also makes you feel fuller and not feel too hungry between meals.

Potatoes

As mentioned earlier, the goal is to consume foods that are filling and can keep you going for hours, one such being potatoes. Potatoes are rich in carbs that can keep you sated for hours. Make sure you either steam and mash them or roast them without the addition of any oil or fat.

Deep frying them is never an option. Try to consume them with their skin on as the skin contains a lot of nutrients.

Probiotics

When it comes to digestion, both your liver and gut play a very important role. Both of them need a healthy dose of probiotics in order to function optimally.

If you have an unhealthy gut then you might suffer from side effects such as constipation and even leaky gut syndrome. The best way to combat these is by consuming as many probiotics as possible. Some natural foods rich in probiotics include kombucha and kefir. Add these to your meals and you are sure to experience positive benefits. An alternative is to go for probiotic supplements. Make sure you know which ones to go for. It would be best to consult a physician first.

Assorted Berries

There is nothing better than consuming fresh berries in the mornings. They are loaded with antioxidants and vital nutrients required to keep your body healthy. Strawberries, raspberries, blueberries, and gooseberries all are great for you.

Just toss them into the blender with some milk or yogurt to make a smoothie. According to studies, those who consumed berries regularly were able to remain within their ideal body weight and did not gain too much weight over longer periods.

Eggs

An important aspect of losing weight is building lean muscles. Lean muscles replace regular ones and prevent fat from getting stored. The best way to build lean muscle is by consuming foods rich in proteins. One important source of protein is eggs. Those who consume eggs for breakfast are in a better position to develop lean muscles and not go hungry before the next meal.

Eggs can be quite versatile and cooked in any way you like.

Hard-boil them the previous day so that you have a ready meal the next morning. Simply toss them in a pan to scramble them. It only takes a few minutes to cook them.

Whole Grains

One aspect of maintaining a clean and healthy diet is going for whole grains. The intermittent fast promotes consumption of these, as they are easier for the body to digest and keep the system clean. They are also loaded with proteins and fiber. Do not limit yourself to the usual such as wheat and oats and go for something different such as Bulgar, amaranth, and flax.

Legumes

If you wish to remain full for longer and not feel hungry or peckish too often then there is nothing better than legumes and beans. These cannot only be quite flavorful but also loaded with fiber. The body does not easily digest fiber. In fact, the body cannot digest it at all but makes an extra effort in trying to digest it thereby drawing into the fat reserves. It is, therefore, best to load up on fiber in order to lose weight easily. There are many options to pick from including peas, lentils, green beans, fava, black-eyed peas, etc. These easily fit into soups and salads.

Nuts

Nuts are fatty no doubt, but they contain good fat. Not all fat is bad fat as there can be some good fat as well. Polyunsaturated fats are said to be good for the body and can keep you feeling full for longer. You will not feel hungry if you munch on some walnuts or almonds. But make sure you make them a part of your meal and do not snack on them. Snacking on them can leave you feeling full and disrupt your meal plan. Do not worry about the calorie aspect. Nuts are not as calorific as you may have thought. They contain far fewer calories than some of the other fatty foods that people tend to snack on.

These happen to be superfoods that you must include in your diet while you take up intermittent fasting.

PART 3: MEAL PLAN

CHAPTER 13
THE 14-DAY GROCERY LIST

Meal prep might seem a bit challenging at first but just remember—you don't need to prep all of your meals at one time. You can begin with the meats one evening and veggies the next; it's all up to you! The segment using veggies in this book are prepared to use within a couple of days (unless otherwise shown). Decide How to Prep: Do you want to prepare all of the chicken, pork, or other meal selections one night and the veggies the next night? Or: Do you want to cook each meal individually but in bulk? No worries, either way, since each of the recipes has instructions for individual prep tips as well.

Purchase the containers you want to use. These are some guidelines for those:

- Mason Jars – Pint or quart size
- Ziploc-type freezer bags

- Rubbermaid Stackable – Glad Containers
- Microwavable
- Freezer Safe
- Stackable
- BPA Free
- Reusable

Label the Containers: There are some other things you have to consider when freezing your meals. You should always label your container with the date that you put it in the freezer. You also need to double-check that your bottles, jars, or bags are each sealed tightly. If your containers aren't air-tight, your food will become freezer burnt and need to be trashed.

Set Aside Quiet Time for Prep Day: Choose a time when you won't have any interruptions.

Inventory the Kitchen: Buy your food in bulk to reduce the cost. Saving money while on the ketogenic diet is vital. Purchasing your items in bulk can make a severe impact. Check your area for local farms that raise their animals on pasture feeding or a local market for fresh produce. After you find a good deal, stock up and purchase pantry items such as seasonings and flour. You can freeze many things and save a bundle of cash.

Select Your Meal Plan: You will begin with your 30-day plan and build from there. As you proceed with your daily selections, make notes of which ones you enjoyed the most and the ones you want to omit for your next month's planning.

Chop your veggies in advance: Prepare and freeze plenty of healthy fruits and yogurt into a delicious smoothie for the entire week. Enjoy one for breakfast or any time you have the craving.

Purchase foods in bulk to be used for taco meats, breakfast burritos, fajita fillings, soups, egg muffins, and so much more. As you prep, include lean proteins for the weekends in a container for a quick grab 'n' go snack or luncheon for a weekend journey.

Tips for Vegetable & Meat Selections

Select fresh meats and dairy when possible – Try to find meat and dairy that has an expiration date for as far in the future as possible. These choices will tend to remain fresh and last longer. This also applies to the "sell by" dates. The further in the future, either of these dates is, the surer you can bet that the food is going to last the week.

Select Whole – Not Chopped Meats & Veggies. You can save big by chopping your own meats and vegetables. You will pay for the person that is doing the cutting for your convenience.

Freeze & Reheat Your Meals – The Healthy Way: For meals that are scheduled to be eaten at least three days after cooking, freezing is a great option. Freezing food is safe and convenient, but it doesn't work for every type of meal. You can also freeze the ingredients for a slow cooker meal and then just dump out the container into the slow cooker and leave it there. This saves a lot of time and means you can pre-prep meals up to 1-2 months in advance.

The last food safety consideration you need to make with regards to meal prepping is how you reheat food. Most people opt to microwave their meals for warming, but you can use any other conventional heating source in your kitchen as well. The reason people love the microwave for heating their meal prep meals is that it's quick and convenient. However, you have to be careful with microwaving because over-cooking can cause food to taste bad. To combat this, cook your food in one minute intervals and check on it between each minute.

You can also help your food cook more evenly and quickly but keeping your meat cut into small pieces when you cook it. You should never put frozen food directly from the freezer into the microwave. Let your frozen food thaw first. Food reheating and prep safety will become second nature over time. Meal prep is challenging when you are just starting out but become much simpler after you have seen it done. There are also errors that can be avoided. However, mistakes do happen, and as such, it's best to cook for short periods of time rather than longer ones, so you have less of a risk of making a mistake and needing to scrap everything you have prepared for that substantial period of time. While it is a lot and seems complicated, meal prepping is the best way to set yourself up for success with the keto diet.

Example of How Meal Prep Works – The Shopping List

- Choose Healthy Produce: Carrots, red bell peppers, cucumbers, baby spinach, and any other keto-friendly veggies you prefer.

- Protein Options: Two cans of tuna, one pound of lunch meat of your choice (turkey, ham, roast beef), and two pounds of skinless chicken thighs or one pound of salmon (this will be used for lunch and dinner)
- Dairy Options: Cheese sticks (of your choice), heavy cream, sour cream, grass-fed butter, keto-friendly salad dressing, mayo, mustard, and eggs.
- Dry Goods Options: Coffee, avocado oil, pecans, almonds, salt, pepper, and your seasonings of choice

Method of Preparation

From there, you will do the following steps to prepare your lunch and dinner for the week:

- Get ten plastic containers ready to fill with your meals.
- Chop up vegetables and put them in five different plastic containers.
- Combine baby spinach salad with vegetables of choice to make five salads.
- Boil eggs and peel.

- Mix the canned tuna with mayo, mustard, salt, and pepper. Put the tuna salad in two different plastic containers that already have a salad or mixed vegetables in them.
- Bake four pieces of chicken and four pieces of salmon. Season it with your seasonings of choice and cook them in avocado oil.
- Combine four pieces of salmon and four pieces of chicken with the ten containers that are already filled with salad and chopped vegetables.
- Finish the ten meals by adding your choice of pecans, almonds, hard-boiled eggs, and cheese sticks. These will be snacks to supplement your meals.

You are ready to go and prepared all of your breakfast, lunch, and dinner for the coming week. This method takes two to three hours and provides well-balanced meals for each of the seven nights of the week.

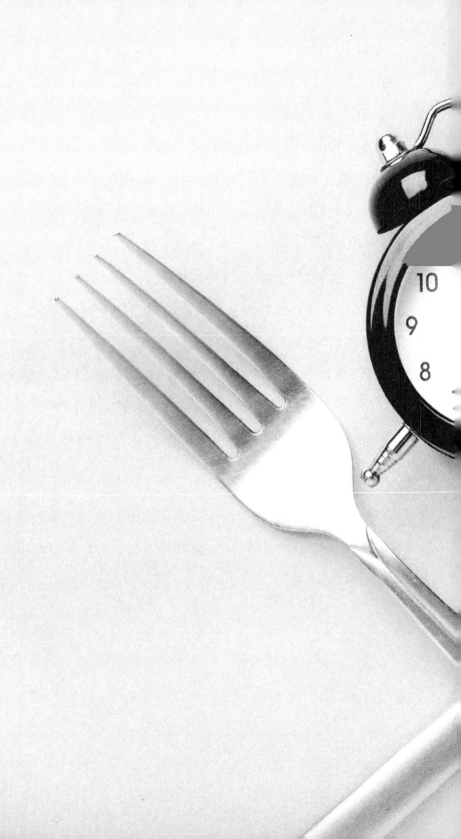

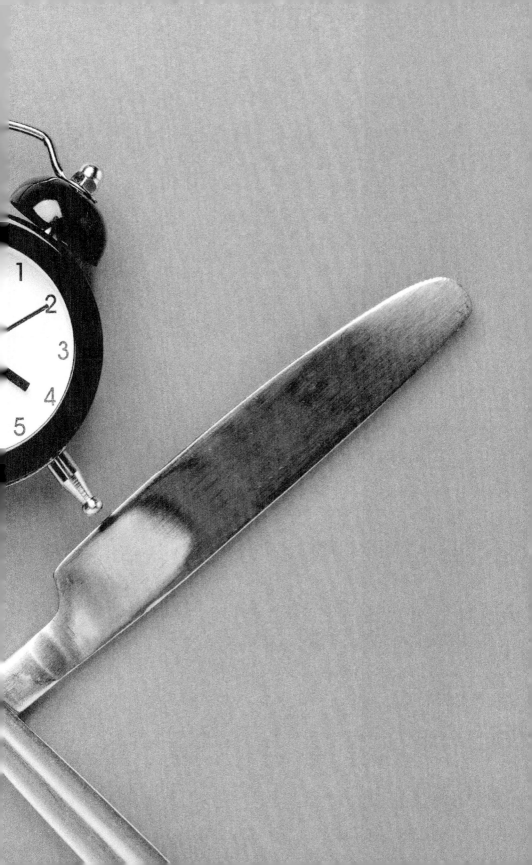

CHAPTER 14
THE 14-DAY RECIPES

BREAKFAST

1 Smoked Salmon Omelet

Preparation Time: 5-10 min.

Cooking Time: 20 min.

Difficulty: Easy

Servings: 1

Ingredients:

- 2 medium eggs
- Smoked salmon, sliced
- Rocket, chopped
- 1/2 teaspoon capers
- 1 teaspoon Parsley, chopped
- 1 teaspoon extra virgin olive oil

Directions:

1. Break the eggs in a bowl and stir well.
2. Add the salmon, capers, parsley and rocket.
3. In a non-stick frying pan, heat the olive oil until hot but not smoking.
4. Add the egg mixture and move the mixture around the pan, using a spatula or fish slice, until it is even.
5. Reduce fire and let cook through the omelet.
6. Stir spatula around the edges and roll the omelet up or fold in half to serve.

Nutrition:

- Calories: 288.1
- Fat: 30 g
- Protein: 56 g
- Carbohydrate: 0 g
- Cholesterol: 230 mg
- Sugar: 0 g

2 Mushroom Scramble Egg

Preparation Time: 5 min.

Cooking Time: 10 min.

Difficulty: Easy

Servings: 3

Ingredients:

- 2 eggs
- 1 teaspoon ground turmeric
- 1 teaspoon mild curry powder
- 20g kale, roughly chopped
- 1 teaspoon extra virgin olive oil
- ½ bird's eye chili, thinly sliced
- A handful of thinly sliced, button mushrooms
- 5 g parsley, finely chopped

Directions:

1 Mix the curry and turmeric powder, then add a little water until a light paste has been achieved.
2 Steam up the kale for 2-3 minutes.
3 At medium heat, heat the oil in a frying pan and fry the chili and mushrooms for 2-3 minutes till they start browning and softening.
4 Put the eggs and spice paste, and cook over medium heat, then add the kale and start cooking for another minute over medium heat. Add the parsley, then mix well and serve.

Nutrition:

- Calories: 182
- Fat: 30 g
- Protein: 76 g
- Carbohydrate: 0 g
- Cholesterol: 130 mg
- Sugar: 0 g

3 **Matcha Green Tea Smoothie**

Preparation Time: 3 min.

Cooking Time: 0 minute

Difficulty: Easy

Servings: 2

Ingredients:

- 2 ripe bananas
- 2 teaspoons matcha green tea powder
- 2 teaspoons honey
- 1/2 teaspoon vanilla bean paste (not extract) or a small scrape of the seeds from a vanilla pod
- 250 ml of milk
- Six ice cubes

Directions:

1 Blend all the ingredients

in a blender and serve in two glasses.

Nutrition:

- Calories: 183
- Fat: 30 g
- Protein: 56 g
- Carbohydrate: 0 g
- Cholesterol: 0 mg
- Sugar: 10 g

4   Date and Walnut Porridge

Preparation Time: 10 min.

Cooking Time: 0 min.

Difficulty: Medium

Servings: 1

Ingredients:

- 200 ml Milk or dairy-free alternative
- 1 teaspoon Walnut butter or four chopped walnut halves
- 1 Medjool date, chopped
- 1.75 ounce of Strawberries, hulled
- 1.45 ounce of Buckwheat flakes

Directions:

1 Place the milk and date in a saucepan, heat gently, then add the buckwheat flakes and cook until the porridge is the consistency you like.
2 Stir in the butter of walnut or walnuts, top with the strawberries and serve.

Nutrition:

- Calories: 183
- Fat: 30 g
- Protein: 56 g
- Carbohydrate: 10 g
- Cholesterol: 230 mg
- Sugar: 0 g

LUNCH

5 Asian Chicken Wings

Preparation Time: 10 min.

Cooking Time: 35 min.

Difficulty: Hard

Servings: 5

Ingredients:

- 2 lbs. chicken wings
- 2 tablespoons sesame oil
- ¼ cup tamari sauce
- 1 tablespoon ginger powder
- 2 teaspoons white wine vinegar
- 3 garlic cloves, minced
- ¼ teaspoon sea salt

Directions:

1. Preheat oven to 400°F.
2. In a large container whisk together the ginger powder, sesame oil, salt, tamari sauce, vinegar, and garlic.
3. Add the wings to the mixture and stir to coat.
4. Place the wings on a lined baking sheet and bake for 30-35 minutes until golden and crispy.
5. If you want it crispier, turn on the broiler for a few minutes. Enjoy!

Nutrition:

- Calories: 277
- Fat: 7 g
- Fiber: 2 g
- Carbs: 8 g
- Protein: 23 g

6 Baked Garlic Ghee Chicken Breast

Preparation Time: 5 min.

Cooking Time: 30 min.

Difficulty: Medium

Servings: 1

Ingredients:

- 1 chicken breast
- 1 teaspoon garlic powder
- 1 tablespoon ghee
- 2 garlic cloves, chopped
- 1 teaspoon sea salt
- 1 teaspoon chives, diced

Directions:

1. Preheat oven to 350°F.
2. Place the chicken breast on a piece of foil.

3. Season with sea salt, garlic powder, chopped fresh garlic.
4. Top with ghee and rub everything into the chicken breast.
5. Wrap the chicken breast in the foil and place it on a baking tray.
6. Bake for 30 minutes, or until chicken breast is cooked through, with a meat thermometer reading above 165°F.
7. Serve with more salt and ghee to taste. Cut the chicken breast into slices and sprinkle diced chives on top.

Nutrition:

- Calories: 264
- Fat: 15 g
- Fiber: 2 g
- Carbs: 6 g
- Protein: 24 g

7 Lamb Curry

Preparation Time: 10 min.

Cooking Time: 4 hours

Difficulty: Medium

Servings: 6

Ingredients:

- 2 tablespoons fresh ginger, grated
- 2 garlic cloves, peeled and minced
- 2 teaspoons cardamom
- 1 onion, peeled and chopped
- 6 cloves
- 1 pound lamb meat, cubed
- 2 teaspoons cumin powder
- 1 teaspoon garam masala
- ½ teaspoon chili powder
- 1 teaspoon turmeric
- 2 teaspoons coriander
- 1-pound spinach
- 14 ounces canned

Directions:

1. In a slow cooker, mix lamb with tomatoes, spinach, ginger, garlic, onion, cardamom, cloves, cumin, garam masala, chili, turmeric, and coriander.
2. Stir well. Cover and cook on high for 4 hours.
3. Uncover the slow cooker, stir the chili, divide into bowls, and serve.

Nutrition:

- Calories: 186
- Fat: 7 g

- Fiber: 2 g
- Carbs: 8 g
- Protein: 26 g

8 Healthy Baby Carrots

Preparation Time: 10 min.

Cooking Time: 20 min.

Difficulty: Easy

Servings: 4

Ingredients:

- 1 lb. baby carrots
- 1 teaspoon Italian seasoning
- 1 tablespoon balsamic vinegar
- 2 tablespoons olive oil
- 1/4 cup vegetable stock
- Pepper
- Salt

Directions:

1. Add all ingredients into the inner pot of the Instant Pot and stir well.
2. Seal pot with lid and cook on high for 20 minutes.
3. Once done, allow to release pressure naturally for 5 minutes then release remaining using quick release. Remove lid.
4. Serve and enjoy.

Nutrition:

- Calories: 105
- Fat: 7.5 g
- Carbs: 9.6 g
- Protein: 0.8 g

Emma Vogel

DINNER

9 Garlic Bread Stick

Preparation Time: 10 min.

Cooking Time: 20 min.

Difficulty: Medium

Servings: 4

Ingredients:

- ¼ cup butter softened
- 1 tsp. garlic powder
- 2 cups almond flour
- ½ tbsp. baking powder
- 1 tbsp. Psyllium Husk® powder
- ¼ tsp. salt
- 3 tbsp. butter, melted
- 1 egg
- ¼ cup boiling water

Directions:

1. Preheat your oven to 400°F/200°C. Line a baking sheet with parchment paper and keep it on the side.
2. Beat the butter with garlic powder and keep it on the side. Add the almond flour, baking powder, husk, salt in a bowl and mix in the butter and egg; mix well.
3. Pour the boiling water into the mixture and stir until you have a nice dough. Divide the dough into 8 balls and roll into breadsticks.
4. Place on a baking sheet and bake for 15 minutes. Brush each stick with the garlic and butter and bake for 5 more minutes. Serve and enjoy!

Nutrition:

- Calories: 259
- Fats: 24 g
- Carbs: 5 g
- Protein: 7 g

10 Steam Your Own Lobster

Preparation Time: 10 min.

Cooking Time: 10 min.

Difficulty: Medium

Servings: 4

Ingredients:

- 4 lobster tails
- 1 sprig parsley

Directions:

1. If the lobster tails are frozen, defrost them.
2. Before cooking, make a long slit in the underbelly of the lobster.
3. Fill a pot halfway with water. Place a steamer basket inside.
4. Once the water is boiling, place the lobster tails onto the steamer attachment.
5. Let boil for 8-9 minutes for fresh lobster and 10 minutes for defrosted lobster.
6. Garnish with parsley.

Tip: If using fresh lobster, steam it for 8-9 minutes.

Nutrition:

- Calories: 100
- Protein: 24 g

11 Garlic Ghee Pan-Fried Cod

Preparation Time: 5 min.

Cooking Time: 10 min.

Difficulty: Easy

Servings: 4

Ingredients:

- 1¼ lb. cod fillets
- 3 tbsps. ghee
- 6 garlic cloves, minced
- 1 tbsp. garlic powder
- A pinch salt

Directions:

1. In a frying pan over medium-high heat, melt the ghee.
2. Add half of the minced garlic.
3. Place the cod fillets in the pan and sprinkle with garlic powder and salt.
4. Cook until the cod fillets are a solid white color, about 4-5 minutes.
5. Then flip the cod fillets and add the remaining minced garlic. Cook until the whole fillets turn a solid white color, about 4-5 minutes.
6. Serve with the ghee and garlic from the pan.

Nutrition:

- Calories: 160
- Carbs: 1 g
- Fats: 7 g
- Protein: 21 g

SNACKS

12 Orange and Apricot Bites

Preparation Time: 10 min.

Cooking Time: 10 min.

Difficulty: Easy

Servings: 4

Ingredients:

- ¾ cup coconut
- ½ cup almond butter
- ½ cup dried apricots
- 1 ½ cups pitted dates
- 1 cup oats, toasted
- 1 tsp. vanilla
- 3 tbsps. Orange juice
- 1 tbsp. orange zest

Directions:

1. Preheat the oven to 350°F/180°C and line some parchment paper on a baking sheet.
2. Place the oats on the baking sheet and toast them for a few minutes until they are slightly toasted.
3. While your oats are in the oven, take out the food processor and add in the dates. Pulse until smooth.
4. Add the vanilla, orange juice and zest, coconut, almond butter, apricots, and toasted oats to the food processor.
5. Pulse so that the mixture gets a smooth consistency. Transfer the mixture into a bowl.
6. Use your hands to make little balls out of the batter and place them into a resealable container. Allow these to set for at least 15 minutes and then serve.

Nutrition:

- Calories: 117
- Fats: 2 g
- Carbs: 17 g
- Protein: 3 g

13 Zucchini Chips

Preparation Time: 35 min.

Cooking Time: 25 min.

Difficulty: Easy

Servings: 4

Ingredients:

- 1 lb. organic zucchini
- 1/3 cup olive oil

- Unrefined sea salt, to taste

Directions:

1. Trim the ends of zucchini and slice them thinly. Toss the zucchini slices in a bowl with olive oil and salt.
2. Place the zucchini slices on a microwave-safe plate and cook for 10 minutes uncovered.
3. Check the chips, and then cook for a few more minutes, until crispy. You can also cook these in a toaster oven, on low heat for a longer amount of time, up to an hour.
4. Allow the chips to cool and then serve with a low-carb dip or dressing of your choice. Enjoy!

Nutrition:

- Calories: 80
- Fats: 6 g
- Saturated Fats: 1.5 g
- Cholesterol: 5 mg
- Sodium: 320 mg
- Carbs: 4 g
- Sugar: 3 g
- Fiber: 1 g
- Protein: 3 g

14 Calamari Rings

Preparation Time: 5 min.

Cooking Time: 2 min.

Difficulty: Easy

Servings: 4

Ingredients:

- 4 calamari squid tubes
- 1 tbsp. ghee
- 2 tbsp. almond flour
- 1 lemon, juiced and zested
- Salt and pepper, to taste

Directions:

1. Mix almond flour, lemon zest, salt, and pepper.
2. Slice the squid tubes into ½-inch slices.
3. Roll the calamari rings in the almond mix.
4. Heat the ghee in a frying pan and fry the rings over low heat for 1 minute on each side until cooked and golden.
5. Drizzle with lemon juice.

Nutrition:

- Calories: 159
- Carbs: 5.9 g
- Fats: 8.2 g
- Protein: 16.3 g

Conclusion

Thank you for reading through to the end of Intermittent Fasting for Women after 50. By now, you must've found this book to be extremely helpful in providing you with all of the resources you need to accomplish your health and longevity goals, whatever they might look like for you.

Now, the next step in your health journey is to move further and decide on a plan you'll follow that can catapult you to a higher degree of success. If you do need assistance getting underway, you'll probably get great results by first reviewing your daily diet and exercise routine before deciding on a feasible intermittent fasting regimen.

Remember, you're not bettering your health for others; you're doing it for your future self. Intermittent fasting is a fantastic way to schedule meal hours, not just for losing fat but also for leading a healthy, vibrant lifestyle that has many health benefits. Considering how busy life is for women of any age, intermittent fasting, specifically for older women, is unlike all the other weight-loss plans, which are either very hard to follow every day consistently, are costly, and produce just modest results. Intermittent fasting is both free and quick to enforce. Simply alter your dietary habits such that you alternate times of fasting with periods of feasting. This book is a particularly valuable guide for helping you during the adjustment to a new way of life. Know you don't have to alter your diet; alternatively, adopt a different form of eating that suits your lifestyle. In fact, you could still carry on with your exercise program even though you'll have to customize it to the existing scenario in contexts of when you consume food and how intense your gym sessions are.

So, what exactly are you looking for? Start planning for your intermittent fasting journey now to enjoy the rewards. Use the knowledge you've gained from this book as a launching pad to get ready for and change your life. Of course, a healthy lifestyle has many forms: it doesn't look the same for everyone. Intermittent fasting is just one of the many amazing options people have to better one's health. The most essentials and central tenets of any good lifestyle are still going to be consuming natural, organic food, staying active, and improving your sleep quality. Intermittent fasting can be challenging in the beginning. So if intermittent is not your cup of tea even after trying hard, then you can surely keep looking for the lifestyle that best suits your life and goals and is feasible for you. Because when all is said and done, there is no one-size-fits-all diet or lifestyle when it comes to your longevity and fitness. The best plan is the one that you can sustain for a lifetime. Consistency is everything in life. If you feel at your best during your fasts and find it to be a maintainable way of living, it can be like magic for you to lose weight and improve your health.

Printed in Great Britain
by Amazon